SCALES OF JUSTICE

Exploring the Wilderness of Health Care and Society's Moral Conscience

Emerita T. Gueson, M.D.

Wyndham Hall Press

SCALES OF JUSTICE
Exploring the Wilderness of Health Care and Society's Moral Conscience

by Emerita T. Gueson, M.D.

Wyndham Hall is an academic imprint of the Cloverdale Corporation.

Library of Congress Catalog Card Number

92-050204

International Standard Book Number

1-55605-204-9 softback
1-55605-205-7 hardback

Printed in the United States of America

Cloverdale Corporation
Bristol, IN 46507-9460

To God, whose inspiration, divine intervention, and enlightening guidance have allowed me to see beyond the signs and symptoms of a disease in a patient in order to know the whole person as a dignified human being with spiritual, emotional, psychological, social, and physical needs.

ACKNOWLEDGMENTS

I am thankful to my niece, Jozelle, for typing, editing, and proof-reading the manuscript.

I am particularly grateful to Laurie Guiniven for helping me edit, re-edit, and proofread the manuscript and for her feedback on how the manuscript can best be understood by laymen.

I am thankful and honored that Dr. Ronald Bronow agreed to review the manuscript and write the introduction of the book in spite of a very busy schedule which includes traveling around the country in his efforts to educate the public about the PHYSICIANS WHO CARE TEN POINT PLAN TO SAVE AMERICA'S HEALTH CARE SYSTEM.

INTRODUCTION

"The HMO horror stories described by Dr. Gueson are true. Before you join any of these plans, please read this information provided by Physicians Who Care. HMO's consistently 'neglect' to inform prospective patients of these facts." If you are thinking of joining an HMO consider the following...

Q. "What is an HMO?"

A. An HMO (Health Maintenance Organization) is a group, usually a profit-oriented corporation, that contracts with medical facilities, physicians, employers, and sometimes individual patients to provide "complete" medical care to a group of individuals. This care is provided at a fixed price per patient, and the employer usually pays most of this. The medical care is usually made available to patients without a significant out-of-pocket expense.

Q. "This HMO option sounds like a great deal. Nothing out-of-pocket. What's the catch?"

A. You're right. There is a catch. The catch comes in terms of rationing of health care services to you under the plan. An HMO is usually a for-profit organization with responsibility to its stockholders that is placed between you and your physician. The HMO directly or indirectly controls the amount of health care that can be rendered to you by the physician. At times, the "overmanagement" of the health care dollar by an HMO can lead to a frustrating experience for both the patient and physician when working through a medical problem.

Q. "I've been going to my doctor for a long time and he knows me very well. Likewise, I know and trust him. If I change my standard medical insurance to an HMO, can I continue to go to him?"

A. Probably not. Unless your personal physician happens to be a member of the particular HMO you are joining, you can no longer see him or her under the terms of the plan. We feel the physician-patient relationship is something that should span years and not change each time there is a change in employment or a change in the type of insurance coverage your employer selects for a given year. Over the years, your personal physician comes to know you and your family well, including your health, social, and personal problems. This type of long-term relationship is likely to result in a high quality of medical care for you and your family. Changing physicians each time your health care coverage changes interrupts the long-term continuity of care that is so important.

Q. "My physician is a member of the HMO my employer is offering. They are also offering traditional insurance. Shouldn't I just sign up for the HMO since my doctor is a member?"

A. Even if you have a longstanding and satisfactory relationship with your personal physician, once you are a patient in an HMO, you may find an entirely different relationship under the restrictions of the plan. If your physician is a specialist, you probably cannot continue seeing this doctor at all. Many HMO's require you to choose a primary care doctor, usually a family practitioner, from their list. The physician, often called a "gatekeeper", controls your access to medical care within the plan. You cannot go to a specialist, unless the physician feels the medical problem is out of his or her realm of expertise. In many HMO plans, your "gatekeeper" physician may actually be financially penalized for sending you to a specialist, ordering a sophisticated diagnostic test, or allowing you to be seen in the emergency room. This is a critical flaw in the "gatekeeper" controlled HMO. Many primary care physicians in these HMO's find themselves in the difficult position of trying to provide good care to you while burdened with the health care rationing restrictions of the HMO plan. Due to these frustrations, your physicians may not elect to stay on with the HMO plan over the long-term. You may again find yourself starting all over again with another physician on the HMO list.

Q. "We prefer to receive all our care at a particular hospital we have been using for years. Can we still go there if I join an HMO?"

A. It depends on the plan, but be aware that many HMO's limit you to selected hospitals where they have arranged discounts. If your hospital of choice is not on their list, you're out of luck. If for some reason, you wish to receive medical care outside of your area, be prepared for some red tape. You will probably find the HMO will not pay for it unless the situation fits their definition of an emergency, which may be quite different from yours. This is another example of restriction of your access to medical care that you should understand.

Q. "What's your suggestion for avoiding these problems with health care coverage?"

A. We feel traditional health insurance plans provide the optimum coverage for the following reasons:

- Virtually all physicians will accept these insurance plans.
- Virtually all hospitals, anywhere in the country, will accept these insurance plans. If you need health care coverage away from home, these plans will usually cover your expenses and you will avoid a significant amount of red tape in the process.
- If you change employment or insurance plan, as long as you stay with one of these standard traditional health insurance plans, you can continue to see the physician of your choice and use the hospital of your choice.
- Although most private practice physicians are very conscious of medical costs, with traditional health insurance, your doctor can make unbiased medical decisions, assuring you get the care you deserve.
- You will find that any out-of-pocket expense is well worth it in the long run. Remember, you get what you pay for.

Q. "My enrollment for medical coverage comes up soon. I am being asked to choose between HMO, a PPO (Preferred Provider Organization), and standard "80/20" medical insurance. What's the best way to make this decision?"

A. We suggest that you consult your personal physician regarding his or her opinion of the various plans. Doctors know a lot about health care coverage because they see it from the inside. Be cautious of signing up for plans simply because there's no out-of-pocket expense, unless you fully understand the health care rationing and restricted access to medical care in many of these plans. Your personal physician is your advocate in health care and can assist you in determining the true substance of the various options offered to you.

HMO CHECKLIST

These are questions that may help you evaluate HMO's:

- How many subscribers do you have in your area?
- How many primary care physicians are now participating?
- With what companies have you actually contracted?

- Are all participating physicians board certified?
- Do your primary care practitioners have more than one year of training?

- Must all referrals first have approval of the primary care physician?
- Do you use the "gatekeeper" concept to control medical costs? If so, can the "gatekeeper" physician be financially penalized for referring me for specialty consultation, sophisticated diagnostic tests, or an emergency visit? Are there other economic incentives for the physician to limit these types of services to me?
- What recourse do I have if my primary care physician refuses to make a referral?

ACCESS TO SPECIALIZED CARE

- Are all specialties covered?
- What if I need a non-participating specialist?
- Can I continue going to a gynecologist, cardiologist, or other specialist whom I have seen for years and who knows my case history?
- Would I ever be required to see a specialist outside my own geographic area?
- If your participating specialist is not considered the best person for the job, can I see a non-participating physician?

- I want to go to a doctor who does not belong to the HMO. He charges the same fee that HMO would pay; can I be reimbursed?
- If I want second opinion, will HMO pay for it?
- If my HMO doctor and I disagree over medical treatment, what are my options?
- What can I do if my physician wants to send me home from the hospital too soon?

- Will I see a physician each time I come to the clinic?
- Will I see the same physician each time?
- To what extent are nurses or other non-physicians substituted for physicians in the delivery of health care in the HMO?
- What do I do if I need to talk to my doctor after hours? Will I have to plead my case to a triage nurse before I can speak to a physician?
- In some areas, there are reports of long delays in getting appointments for routine visits. How long will I have to wait?

EMERGENCY CARE IN AN HMO

- What do I do in an emergency?
- Am I limited to a particular emergency room?
- Do I have to call the HMO "triage nurse" before I can go to the emergency room?
- What is your definition of an emergency?
- What happens if I disagree?
- In an emergency, if I go to a non-participating hospital emergency room, could there be a delay in my care while the emergency room is trying to reach the HMO by phone for authorization?
- What happens if the HMO refuses to authorize the emergency room visit?
- What if I become ill while I am away from home and it is not an emergency?

COSTS

- How much is the co-payment or deductible?
- Is the amount constant, even on weekends, holidays, and nights?
- Is there a higher co-payment for emergency services or other services?
- If my physician wants to check me briefly to follow up a problem, must I pay another co-payment?
- Am I really saving money by selecting an HMO instead of traditional health insurance? If so, are the restrictions worth it?

HOSPITALS

- Will I be limited to a particular hospital/s?
- Will the HMO pay for ambulance transportation to the hospital?

WHAT IS COVERED/WHAT ISN'T.........THE "FINE PRINT"

- What kind of services or treatment will you not cover?
- Do you provide rehabilitative services in the event of an accident or chronic illness?
- Does your plan pay for organ transplants? Which ones?

- How does your plan handle cancer care? Who provides that care?
- How does your plan handle respiratory diseases? Who provides that care?
- How does your plan handle care for people with heart disease? Who provides that care? Who performs the necessary surgery?
- Does your plan cover mental health care? How much of the counseling is done by non-psychiatrists? How difficult is it to actually see the psychiatrist? How many psychiatrists are available? How many non-psychiatrist counselors are working under this physician?
- Does your plan cover alcohol or drug abuse treatment?
- Does your plan cover allergy treatment?
- What about plastic surgery procedures? Which ones are covered? Who decides whether a particular plastic procedure is medically necessary or elective?
- What recourse do I have if I feel a procedure is medically necessary?
- Will the HMO pay for outpatient physical therapy?
- Will the HMO cover infertility testing and treatment?

DRUGS

- Are HMO patients limited to selected pharmacies?
- Is it true that participating pharmacies will only dispense a limited supply of drugs?
- Are the physicians limited to a fixed formulary of drugs they can prescribe from?

- How are your surplus funds and profits distributed?
- Who oversees the quality of care of the HMO?
- What are the most frequent complaints? Can I see a log of those complaints?

- If I am unhappy with the plan, can I drop out at any time, or am I locked in for a given period?
- What is the dropout rate for subscribers?
- How many physicians have left the plan in the last two years?
- What is the difference between an HMO and a PPO?

- What is covered and under what circumstances if one spouse is in an HMO and the other has another type of health insurance?
- Since the HMO is a group plan, what happens if I am laid off? If I change jobs and my new employer does not have an HMO, will my new insurer make me wait 30-90 days before picking me up?

Traditional health insurance plans give your doctor the greatest flexibility in making decisions about your health. It gives you access to the broad spectrum of medical technology and freedom of choice of physicians and hospitals anywhere in the country.

Physicians Who Care is a national organization of over three thousand physicians and twelve thousand patients who belong to Patients Who Care. Our purpose is to preserve quality medicine and our patients' rights within an environment of cost-cutting. Our patients are sent regular informational pamphlets about important health care issues. They are given the opportunity to inform the media and their elected representatives of their views.

The Physicians Who Care plan on financing health care for the United States has received tremendous attention. Patients all over the country are writing their Senators and Congressmen supporting our ideas. I presented our plan in testimony before the U.S. House of Representatives Ways and Means Committee on March 4th, 1992. For your information I have summarized the ten basic points in the Physicians Who Care proposal.

PHYSICIANS WHO CARE'S TEN POINT PLAN TO SAVE AMERICA'S HEALTH CARE SYSTEM

1. Community rate health insurance so that insurance companies can't insure only the healthy and exclude those with pre-existing illnesses.
2. Provide mandatory employer-sponsored major medical and catastrophic health insurance for all, with the same tax benefits and coverage for the self-insured. Make deductibles high enough to discourage overuse of medical care for minor illnesses, so insurance will be used for serious and catastrophic illnesses only.
3. Set up "Medi-save" accounts using patients' pre-tax dollars to pay for minor illnesses. This leaves minor medical decisions to patients and their physicians rather than to insurance companies.
4. Separate long-term care from Medicaid, so we'll have enough money to care for the poor. Address the problem of long-term care as part of an overall solution.
5. Protect Medicare from the budget cutters by beginning to privatize the program and by allowing Medical IRA accounts.
6. Eliminate state mandated benefits.
7. Allow physicians to develop guidelines for care to protect the public from unnecessary procedures and to allow us physicians to practice quality medicine.
8. Don't force physicians and their patients into for-profit HMO's where the rights of the patients come second to the profit of the corporations.
9. Learn from the impending collapse of the Canadian health care system that government-run medical care is not the answer to our problems.

10. Educate the public so that they will understand that we must all pay for high technology and high quality health care, and that cost containment efforts must not destroy the quality of American medicine.

If you wish more information about our plan, Physicians Who Care or Patients Who Care, please call our national office at 1-800-545-9305.

Ronald Bronow, M.D.

PREFACE

The book measures society's conscience and addresses urgent healthcare issues. It is a morality play. It is an insightful, panoramic view of life and its aspects: parent-child relationships, marital values, dedication to homelife and profession, man's potential in the face of death, loyalty to friends, and the miracle of life. Through it all, it depicts justice, fairness, love, caring, and compassion. It examines the whole healthcare crisis with a view towards finding a possible solution.

Through the creation of fictionalized characters and events, it intimately details how the players of the healthcare revolution, the doctors, the lawyers, the government, the insurance industry, the employers, the healthcare entrepreneurs, and the patients, affect the delivery and quality of healthcare.

It narrates with vivid and almost true-to-life examples how patients are victimized by a profit-motivated and cruel healthcare system. It portrays how the failure of flawed healthcare policies victimizes patients and selectively discriminates against physicians and hospitals. It eloquently illustrates how an unfair legal system abuses both patients and doctors through frivolous medical malpractice suits.

The medical profession itself is helpless and unable to protect its patients because it is besieged by the demands of the government, healthcare insurances, lawyers, and consumers. Through dramatic vignettes, the book illustrates that patients are short-changed because the medical profession has not stood up against the interference of outside forces. It shows how physicians have failed the public in the quest for affordable and accessible quality care for everyone. It shows how lives are lost needlessly through cost-containment. Furthermore, the patients who are most affected in this healthcare crisis are constantly kept in the dark about the medical profession. Conspiracy of silence among physicians is alive and well!

In addition, the book also exposes politicians' driving interest in cutting the federal budget deficit at the expense of the health of patients who feel that these same politicians are genuinely concerned about them. Naively and unknowingly, the elderly, the poor, and the uninsured have fallen through the cracks of cost-containment because of flawed government healthcare policies.

The novel also takes the reader to the world of diseases. It shows, through scenes in the emergency room, intensive care unit, and delivery room, how patients live with disease and how an unexpected disaster can emotionally affect and ruin a family when failure of surgery or treatment occurs.

This novel also takes the reader to the world of physicians when one of the major characters becomes a victim of the system. It tackles the controversial issue of AIDS when a caring physician is infected. It shows the failure of the medical profession to one of its own and poignantly illustrates the lack of compassion that, unfortunately, accompanies the disease because of the ignorance not only of the public, but also of the healthcare workers themselves. This is an issue which needs to be addressed immediately on a national level in order to protect the patients' interests. Also, any healthcare worker afflicted with AIDS because he cared for an AIDS patient needs to be taken care of, too, through healthcare benefits and disability insurance. Every hospital in the country should have its own policy on how to take care of an healthcare worker afflicted with AIDS.

A thoughtful reader will become more puzzled after reading this book. He will realize that the problems affecting the delivery of healthcare is multifaceted. The solution to the healthcare crisis is practically insurmountable! It not only involves economic and budgetary restraints.

It involves moral, ethical, and social issues as well. We have to strengthen our broken-down family unit; otherwise, we will see more teenagers involved in drugs which is draining the resources of emergency rooms. Pregnancy and sexually transmitted diseases are on the rise among the teenage population; obviously, artificial contraception is not the answer to these problems. Abortion has become a form of contraception! The American College of Obstetrics and Gynecology should take a hard look at these problems. Teen star programs for teenagers could be the answer to these problems.

Politicians are dead wrong when they make the pronouncements that hospitals and physicians are the major causes of rising healthcare cost. They should take a hard look at the real issues involved in increasing healthcare cost.

Congress should abolish the financial incentive of HMO's by repealing the Federal HMO Act of 1973. Congress has already passed a law that would make it illegal to have financial incentive on Medicare HMO's. Why, then, is it legal for the rest of regular HMO's? Isn't this double standard? Congress should also stop pushing mandatory generic drug prescriptions to the poor and the elderly, and should repeal the Medicare DRG! The inspector general's office should stop prosecuting doctors for fraud when there is only an error in record keeping with no fraud committed!

The justice department should also stop persecuting doctors who try to educate the public about the financial incentives in HMO's by threatening them with antitrust lawsuits. Consumers should have an organization called, perhaps, "Patients Exploited by Healthcare Insurance," in order to protect themselves from the greed of the insurance companies and to make them accountable for trying to set the trend of medical practice!

I must end by saying that the solution to the healthcare crisis involves cooperation from every member of society. We all should be responsible for our actions.

CHAPTER I

Today is July 8, 1986. Market and Arch Streets are teeming with people. There are a lot of television crews and camera men whose attention is directed towards the Federal Courthouse. It is extremely crowded, and one can see people sitting on the steps of the courthouse just to get a glimpse of the defendant. Even the balconies of the buildings that surround the courthouse are crowded, and practically everyone is carrying a telescope. The traffic in nearby streets is jammed! People have to leave their cars in the middle of the streets. People are oblivious to the sweltering heat, the traffic violations, the fines, the parking tickets, and the risk of their cars being towed. The whole city of Philadelphia is agog! The most celebrated and flamboyant lawyer in town, Robert Smith, is going to be sentenced today for murder, inflicting AIDS on homeless people, drug trafficking, money laundering, and obstruction of justice. Robert Smith was formerly an eminent medical malpractice lawyer until the fateful day of February 17, 1984, when he made the mistake of filing a malicious, frivolous medical malpractice suit against an eminent emeritus surgeon at one of the mecca of medical learning in Philadelphia, Dr. Jay Simmons.

Dr. Jay Simmons was set to retire on June 30, 1983. Five months before, on Jan. 9, 1983, while on his way to an early morning administrative meeting, he met one of his former surgical protegees, Dr. James Dillon. Dr. Dillon was on his way to see a patient in the emergency room. So, Dr. Simmons decided to go with him.

The emergency room, which was located in the MacMillan Building of University Hospital, was bustling with activity. In the hallways and corridors, there were patients on stretchers with open intravenous fluids hanging, some on their way to the operating room, some to the intensive care unit, and some to the coronary care unit.

The Triage area, where patients were screened according to the urgency of medical attention, was crowded. The three nurses who interviewed patients had their hands full: a school bus had overturned, and the twenty students on board had been brought to the Triage center.

Opposite the Triage center was the area where the pastoral counselor was consoling the grieving family of an old man who had just been brought in DOA (Dead On Arrival). His wife was uncontrollably hysterical, but his two daughters had taken the bad news with resignation.

Inside the accident ward, there were five students who were injured and awaiting the arrival of an orthopedic surgeon. In room one, an intubated asthmatic was being monitored and was about to be transferred to the ICU. In room two, a pregnant patient was in active labor, ready to be transferred to the delivery floor. In room three, a croupy two-year-old boy in an oxygen tent was ready to be transferred to the pediatric ICU. The other five rooms were occupied by patients awaiting further medical evaluation for possible admission. In room nine, a 17-year-old boy had just had a steroid injection for bee sting. In room ten, a 22-year old woman, who had just had a miscarriage, was about to be moved to the operating room for dilatation and evacuation.

The patient in room eleven was a 48-year-old white man weighing 250 lbs., with noticeable abdominal distention in spite of his obesity. The senior resident who had called Dr. James Dillon, Dr. Michael Olsire, stated that the abdominal tap was bloody. The cardiac monitor showed sinus tachycardia and no arrhythmia. The patient's nailbeds and palms were pale, his face and eyelids were practically paper white. His nailbeds were cold and clammy. His urine output was decreased. His hemoglobin came back 7.5 grams. He had been given albumin solution to maintain his blood volume, while awaiting the four units of blood that were being typed and crossed.

When this patient was first seen in the accident ward, he gave a very scanty medical history. He had slurred speech to the point of being incoherent. His clothes were very dirty; he was drunk and spaced out. He was also shivering. His blood alcohol level was negative. Drug testing was done. He was brought in by the cops who had found him on the sidewalk across from the oldest hotel in Philadelphia.

During all the exchange and communication of medical information, Dr. Jay Simmons just stood there listening; he did not interview or examine the patient. The blood bank called the emergency room, stating that the blood for the patient, Mr. Charlie Singleton (that was the only information available about the patient), had been brought down to the operating room. Three units of blood were pumped. A Swan-Ganz catheter was inserted to monitor the blood volume. The patient was closely monitored by the anesthesiologist. The patient's carbon dioxide and oxygen saturation levels were within normal limits. The patient's abdomen was then prepped and draped. A left paramedian incision was made. The incision was extended into the peritoneal cavity. On opening the peritoneal activity, about 2500 cc of blood was noted. This blood was suctioned. The abdominal retractor (O'Connor-Sullivan) was inserted. An attempt was made to localize the bleeder. The liver was checked, and there was no evidence of lacerations or sources of bleeding. The spleen was inspected, and blood seemed to be oozing from it, but there were no lacerations found! The spleenic vessels were then clamped. The oozing stopped. A splenectomy was done. Hemostasis was then rechecked and accomplished. The patient's abdominal incision was then closed in three layers and dressed. The patient was then watched in the recovery room. Three hours later, he was transferred to the ICU and monitored all night. The patient had an uneventful night. His vital signs (B.P., P.R., R.R.) were stable. He was transferred the next day to room 456. Charlie Singleton had no visitors. The cops who had brought him into the emergency room could not locate his wife and two daughters.

On his second postoperative day, the report of his drug testing came back positive for marijuana. The pathology report came back as rupture of the aberrant vessels of the spleen. Dr. Dillon discussed with Mr. Singleton his psychiatric consultation and referral to a drug rehabilitation center. The patient vehemently refused. He was doing very well surgerywise. On his fourth postoperative day, he disappeared. The nurses looked all over the rooms on the floor, but he could not be found. The security guards were alerted. There was no sign of Mr. Singleton. An incident report was requested. The cops who originally had taken him to the hospital were notified, and they alerted all the cops patrolling the vicinity frequented by the homeless.

At twelve midnight, Dr. Olsire, who was on call the same day Mr. Singleton walked out, was paged STAT for the emergency room. Dr. Olsire, still gasping for breath, came to the accident ward. He had run all the way from the fifth floor of the MacMillan Building since the elevators had broken down. As soon as he came to room 16, he noticed that Mr. Singleton's abdomen was distended and covered with towels. He uncovered the patient's abdomen. The patient's swollen intestines were hanging out of the incision. He immediately instructed the nurses in the operating room to prepare for an emergency surgery. The nurse anaesthetist was notified, who in turn called the anesthesiologist on call. In the course of examining Charlie Singleton, Dr. Olsire noted multiple needle marks on his wrists and arms. He explained to him that, since there was no time to wait for the result of the drug report, he would have to operate with rapid intubation, which meant that Mr. Singleton would have to be intubated awake!

"Are you putting me on? What kind of joke are you trying to tell me?"

"Mr. Singleton, you must realize that your risk of developing complications is very high."

"Tell me about it. I have nothing to look forward to. My life is shot. My wife kicked me out when I started beating up the girls. Don't bother explaining the possible complications. I don't think I will make it."

"Mr. Singleton, it is my responsibility to tell you and to explain to you that you could also develop pneumonia, infections with your incision, urinary tract infection, another wound separation like what you have now, stress ulcer, bowel obstruction, or a blood clot in your lungs that could be life threatening."

The doctor paused and said, "We will be taking you to the operating room shortly. The anesthesiologist will explain to you the risks of anaesthesia."

In twenty minutes, the whole surgical and anaesthesia team was assembled in the operating room. Mr. Singleton was awake during the intubation before general anaesthesia was administered. Two other surgical residents assisted Dr. Olsire. During the procedure, Dr. John Miller accidentally dropped the knife on Dr. Olsire's left hand. Dr. Olsire was furious! Expletive====Another expletive====Expletive!

"How can you do this to me? This patient is high risk for both AIDS and hepatitis. I could be doomed for life because of your carelessness. Now I will have to get tested for hepatitis and AIDS!"

"I'm very sorry; it was an accident."

The closure of the abdomen took longer than usual because of the patient's obesity and markedly swollen tissues.

Mr. Singleton was transferred to the ICU so that he could be monitored closely. Mr. Singleton was having a restful post-operative night.

Code 1 ICU===Code 1 ICU===Code 1 ICU

Everyone ran towards Mr. Singleton's room. Mr. Singleton was having a Gran Mal seizure. One ampule of Sodium Amytal was given. He was maintained on intravenous Valium every four hours.

In his lucid intervals, he asked for his wife and daughters.

"Please, I want to see my wife and daughters. I am sure my wife will feel sorry for me and take me back if she sees me in my present condition. I feel so alone. I envy all these patients whose families come for a visit everyday and every shift. I have no one to talk to, except these drab and faceless walls."

Dr. Olsire came up to see Mr. Singleton in the Intensive Care Unit.

"I heard you kept the night shift on their toes. How do you feel now? Your pulse is strong. Did you get a good night's sleep after your sedation was injected? You look more alert and rested now than in your previous admission. Is there anything I can do for you?"

"Yes, please help me find my wife and two daughters for God's sake! I need them now!"

"I will talk to the social worker as soon as I finish dressing your incision."

Dr. Olsire was getting ready to leave Mr. Singleton's room when he was paged STAT for the Emergency Room. He ran to the Emergency Room as fast as he could, but the patient had expired by the time he got there. He signed the death certificate as Massive Myocardial Infarction. He introduced himself to the deceased's widow and to the two daughters. He was trying to explain to the family the possible cause of Mr. Secula's death, until he finally realized that the man's daughter, Laura, was a surgical resident at a neighboring university hospital. Dr. Olsire's face was as red as an apple. He invited them to have coffee with him at the social spot. After they were done with their coffee, Dr. Olsire walked them out to the parking lot. Everyone was quiet. Laura thanked Dr. Olsire for his kindness.

"What an attractive, lovely blond," thought Dr. Olsire. "I would like to get to know her better."

Dr. Olsire proceeded to the social service department and requested that the police district in the area where Mr. Singleton used to live check to see if his family had moved back to the house.

CHAPTER II

Officer Eagle went to the house of Mr. Singleton. The house was boarded. The neighborhood had been taken over by drug dealers. The streets were dirty. Most of the houses had tall grasses in their lawns. After Officer Eagle looked around, he decided to knock at the third house on Mr. Singleton's block.

A lady with grayish hair, probably in her late fifties, answered the door. She told him that she was very close to Patty Singleton. Then she filled him in on what she knew.

"Patty Singleton and her two daughters have moved in with Patty's widowed mother. Patty and her two daughters have had a very hard life. She's worked all her life. Her husband used to spend all the money he earned on alcohol. She used to work two jobs. He would come home drunk and sometimes would become so violent that his two daughters were scared to death of him. It was a terrible way to live! For them to grow up in a loveless home and in an environment of violence and misery was awful! Michelle and Kathy were basically nice kids and bright students, but both of them failed their senior year! It was so traumatic for them that both tried to commit suicide! Both took an overdose of Darvon compound with alcohol. They had to be hospitalized for ten days at the Detoxification Center of Northend Hospital. After this unfortunate incident, the two girls became wild. Martyr Patty had a hard time dealing with them. I don't know how she kept her sanity!

"Around summertime two years ago, Patty was rushed to the accident ward of a neighboring hospital. Her scalp was split into two after Mr. Singleton threw a portable sewing machine at her head while she was preparing dinner. She had a concussion and was hospitalized for one week. Her husband never showed his face in the hospital. I think Patty made the decision to leave him while she was in the hospital. Their bills were piling up! She could not hack it anymore, even with two jobs. The two girls were also working and promised to help out their mom, but still their earnings were not enough to pay all the monthly bills.

"Patty's decision was hastened when he woke up one night and found her husband trying to forcibly open the bedroom door of their daughters without even knocking!

"I heard Patty say, 'Don't bother my girls! You get out of this house now, and don't ever come back!'

"Her husband said, 'I'm not going anywhere. You can all leave today, and I don't want to see your faces when I come home.'

"Patty ran into the girls' room and stayed there until he left the house. After breakfast, they started packing. Patty called the two places where she worked. She called her mother. She became hysterical while she was telling her what had happened in the last three months. Her mother told her to come live with her.

"Patty rented a U-Haul. They only brought their personal belongings. When they got to her mother's house, her mom was already waiting on her porch. Mrs. Collins ran towards Patty and her grandchildren and hugged them. They unloaded the U-Haul. It didn't take that long to do it. They put all the baggage in the basement and went upstairs to chat and have lunch. It was their first quiet and very inviting lunch in years. For the first time in years, nobody was screaming at them while they were eating!"

The neighbor stopped for a minute, then added, "When the girls were born, the Singleton family was a typical American family. They were closely knit. They lived in a well-maintained house. They went to church on Sundays. They took the kids to the park on weekends, and both sets of in-laws were a regular fixture in the Singleton household. Patty stayed home to take care of the girls. Taking care of the twins was a lot of fun and hard work. Patty used to run four loads of diapers a day. Between diaper changes and feeding two kids simultaneously, she hardly had time left for herself. She didn't care. She wanted to be home while the kids were growing up. The girls were the center of attention in the church, and in the neighborhood. They just looked like two Dresden dolls. The Singletons were very happy. The kids started nursery school when they turned four. Patty took them to school and picked them up after school. She took a part-time job while the kids were in school, but Charlie Singleton didn't want Patty to work.

"'Why do you have to work?' he asked. 'I am making enough money to support all of us.'

"'I'm thinking about the kids' college education. We have to start saving for them and for our retirement.'

"Charlie was in deep thought and said, 'You are probably right. I will have to start helping you with the household chores.'

"'That's fine with me.'

"Years before Charlie started drinking, he and Patty always sat down and were able to discuss their problems. They were never stingy with praise for each other. Their world was in full bloom! Nothing could go wrong, so they thought. It was the thirteenth birthday party for the twins. All the kids in the neighborhood were invited. The twins were getting ready to blow out the candles on their birthday cake when Charlie walked in with an unsteady gait! Patty could not believe what she was seeing. She excused herself from the guests and the children. She grabbed Charlie by the arm and took him upstairs to their bedroom.

"'Charlie, what is wrong? What is going on at work? This is the first time I have seen you in this condition. Please, tell me what is bothering you. I'm your wife!'

"'Well, do you really want to know? I just got laid off! The company went bankrupt. What am I going to do? I don't even have enough pension to withdraw to tide us over until I find another job.'

"'Don't worry, I am going to work full-time while you are looking for a new job. I am going to ask Mom if she can pick up the kids after school.'

"Days, months, and more months passed, but there was no job in sight for Charlie. He became very depressed when their bills started piling up. He would holler at bill collectors whenever they called. There was even an instance when their phone had to be disconnected. Patty used to cover up for her husband; their parents didn't know that Charlie was not working until after he was six months unemployed. Charlie started drinking everytime he got rejected at job interviews. Finally, after one year of not finding a job, he gave up! I don't know how Patty was able to put up with him. He even bought alcohol with the money meant for food and groceries. One snowy Christmas morning, Patty found him lying on the snow-covered street, drunk and practically frozen from nearly zero temperature. She called an ambulance, and he had to be admitted to the hospital; he stayed for two days.

"Patty tried her best to keep the family together. She went with Charlie to an Alcoholic Anonymous meeting. After attending the Al-Non meeting, he refused to go again. Patty was very upset about Charlie's refusal to go back to Al-Non meetings. But, there was nothing she could do! Charlie had to help himself first before anyone could help him.

"After Patty and the girls moved in with her mother, she called me and gave me her new phone number. I am not supposed to give it to anyone. I must ask her permission first. Please give me the number where you can be reached, and I will call you."

"Officer Eagle, 928-0408."

"I am Mrs. Fearless. I will give you my phone number, in case Charlie's condition changes."

"Thank you for the information. I will give this information to the social worker and Dr. Olsire."

As soon as Officer Eagle arrived at his precinct, he called Dr. Olsire. Dr. Olsire was scrubbed in the operating room, and the message was taken by an O.R. nurse. Dr. Olsire did not finish his surgery until very late in the afternoon. By the time he called Officer Eagle, he had gone off for the day. He went up to see Charlie Singleton again.

"Doc, did you find out anything about my family?"

"Not yet. I was scrubbed when Officer Eagle called. I have to call him up tomorrow morning. I will let you know then. Mr. Singleton, I would like to ask you some personal questions. Do you mind?"

"Not at all."

"Where did you get your recreational drugs? Where did you get the money to buy the drugs?"

"Well, when I started this bad habit, it did not cost me anything. A well-dressed, distinguished-looking guy would come and give us coke. After three months, he started charging us. We were so hooked on coke that we had no choice when he started blackmailing us."

"How did he blackmail you?"

"He told us that if we did not sell coke or crack or whatever street drugs he wanted us to sell, he was going to turn us in to the cops."

"And you did not have a choice?"

"No, because we were dealing with a very powerful man. We found out that he was a well-known legal figure in Philadelphia."

"Would you be able to identify him?"

"He is about six-foot-four with dark blue eyes, black hair, and a red birthmark at the nape of his neck."

"Do you ever read about him in the newspapers or hear about him on the radio or see him on television?"

"I think so."

"I hope you will alert me in case you read about him or see him on television."

"I certainly will."

"Is there anything I can do for you today?"

"I can't think of anything. Thank you, Dr. Olsire."

The next morning, Dr. Olsire called Officer Eagle.

Officer Eagle said, "Dr. Olsire, I have the telephone number of Mrs. Singleton. Would you like to call her and tell her what is going on with Mr. Singleton?"

"What is the best time for me to call her?"

"After 6:00 p.m., but before 8:00 p.m. She works two jobs."

Dr. Olsire went to make rounds and spent a few minutes with Charlie Singleton. He told him that he might be able to talk to Patty Singleton tonight.

"I will come back tonight, as soon as I have talked to your wife."

Dr. Olsire called Mrs. Singleton. Patty was very evasive at first, but later she became comfortable talking to Dr. Olsire.

"I don't think I can come and visit Charlie now. I have too many problems I have to deal with. My younger twin, Kathy, got involved with another 18-year-old boy. She met him at the fast food store where she works part-time. They have both been using drugs for about six months now. As if that's not enough, Kathy's pregnant! We have been going to a counselor. I want her to make a decision about giving up the baby for adoption. We have been getting moral and financial support from some pro-life groups. She has been offered an opportunity to live with several unwed mothers at St. Theresa's Home in Bucks County. She almost had an abortion without my knowledge. I am grateful that an Operation Rescue volunteer was able to talk her out of it."

"I am sorry to hear about your family having so many problems. I wish I could help you in some way. Let me know if there is anything I can do for you. Even if you just need someone to listen to you, to help you ventilate your stress and emotions, I will be available."

"How is Charlie? Is he going to be discharged soon? I wish I could take him back, but it is impossible. He and my mother never got along well. Moreover, I do not know how he will take Kathy's present situation. I will try to see him as soon as I have found a solution to Kathy's problems."

"Please keep me posted, and I will try to call you if there is any change with Mr. Singleton's condition."

"Thank you for your time."

Dr. Olsire went back to the surgical floor to talk to Charlie.

"Doc, were you able to talk to Patty?"

"Yes, but she can't come and visit you yet. She is trying to sort out her feelings. It will take a while for her to come to terms with you. Please give her time. I promised her that I would keep her informed of your progress."

"Doc, thank you for your time and effort."

"You are welcome."

The next morning, Dr. Olsire went to the Social Service Department to initiate the application for Charlie Singleton's medical assistance. Once the medical assistance was approved, his social worker could start applying for a boarding home for Charlie or even for a nursing home for custodial care.

Dr. Olsire informed Charlie that he would most probably be transferred to a boarding home, and a visiting nurse would check on him and then report his progress to Dr. Olsire.

After two weeks, Charlie's medical assistance application was approved and arrangements were made for his transfer to a boarding home.

On the day he was supposed to be moved, he started complaining of chest pain.

"Help, help! I can't breathe! My chest is pounding!" Charlie screamed. He had barely gotten the words out of his mouth when he collapsed.

Code 1, Room 201===Code 1, Room 201

Every doctor in sight ran towards Charlie's room. Charlie was finally revived. Dr. Olsire came in running from the operating room, practically out of breath.

"My God, Charlie, can you hear me? How do you feel?"

"I feel like I am going to drown, and my chest, I mean, I feel so much stabbing pain in my chest. Do you think I will make it?"

"I think so. We are going to move you to the ICU. I think you threw a blood clot. We are running intravenous blood thinners now, and I will also check your heart enzymes just to be sure it's not a heart attack. We are going to hook you up to a cardiac monitor, and you will have to keep your oxygen mask on, too. You will not be able to eat for a couple of days. I am going to call your wife."

"Thank you, Doc. You are so good and attentive to my needs."

"Charlie, that's why I'm a doctor. I love talking to people. I love being involved with their problems. It gives me a lot of personal satisfaction knowing that I have made someone comfortable and have eased his personal pains, and maybe have made a difference in his outlook on life. I will see you later."

Michael Olsire called Patty Singleton at home. Her mother answered.

"Patty can't take phone calls at work, unless it is an absolute emergency."

"Mrs. Collins, I swear, this is an absolute emergency."

Mrs. Collins finally relented and gave Patty's work phone number. Dr. Olsire called Patty at work.

"Mrs. Singleton, I am sorry to tell you that Charlie is now in the ICU. He threw blood clots in his lungs. He will have to stay in the ICU for a while. He was getting ready to be transferred to a boarding home. All of a sudden, he collapsed. We are monitoring him very closely. Some of the studies are already back. His cardiac enzymes are normal. The blood gases point to a blood clot. I will order a lung scan as soon as he is stabilized. We have already started him on the blood thinner, Heparin, which he will be on for at least ten days. A chest X-ray was also taken, and it is suggestive of an embolism. Please feel free to call me, if you have any questions. I know how you must feel, but, if you want to come and see Charlie, you can do that anytime. Just identify yourself. Take care."

Patty was dumbfounded and exclaimed, "God, please give me a break! Show me the way."

Dr. Olsire went back to the ICU to tell Charlie Singleton that he was able to talk to Patty. Charlie's face brightened and he smiled.

"Thank you, Doc. I hope Patty visits me soon. I hope she brings my two daughters with her."

"Charlie, I will see you tomorrow. Everything is under control. All the clinical and laboratory data point to pulmonary embolism. You will be on intravenous blood thinners for about ten days; then I will gradually wean you to an oral anticoagulant, Coumadin. Please get a good night's sleep."

"What a caring physician!"

The next morning, Dr. Olsire got a telephone call from Patty Singleton.

"Dr. Olsire, I would like to visit Charlie this afternoon after I get off from work."

"That would be fine. Please have the lady at the information desk page me as soon as you get here. I do not know how Charlie will react. You have not seen each other for two years. Your separation was so bitter. I hope everything will be fine."

"I hope so, too."

"Don't get upset with the infection precautions posted in Charlie's room."

"Thanks for warning me."

CHAPTER III

Early Friday morning, Dr. Olsire received a call from Patty Singleton.

"Dr. Olsire, I have mixed emotions about visiting Charlie. All of a sudden, all the bad feelings I have harbored and repressed about Charlie and our past relationship and all the bitterness we have felt towards each other keep flashing back into my mind. I am a nervous wreck. Do you think I should really see him soon?"

"I can't make the decision for you. I know that you have had a hard life with Charlie in the past, but he needs you right now. You are the only family he has. All of his relatives are deceased. You have to sort out your feelings and let me know early next week. I don't know if it would be wise to bring the twins with you. I don't think it would be a good idea for Charlie to see Kathy in her present physical condition. Let me know when you are ready to visit Charlie. You can always have me paged in the hospital."

"Thank you, Dr. Olsire."

Days and weeks passed. Dr. Olsire did not hear from Patty. He was quite concerned so he called her at work. She had not been in for two weeks. He called Patty at home. Mrs. Collins answered the phone.

"Kathy has been in the hospital for two weeks now. She is six months pregnant and has been having painless bleeding for two weeks. Patty has been staying with her every day. She is on absolute bedrest and, everytime she moves, she bleeds. Her doctor said that she has Placenta Praevia. I hope she is able to hold this pregnancy for several weeks more. Her belly is not that big. Probably, the baby is not growing well because of her bleeding problems."

"I am sorry to hear about Kathy's problem. Please tell Patty I called. And, if there is anything I can do for her, just let me know."

"Thank you, Dr. Olsire. You seem like a nice doctor."

Patty called Dr. Olsire the next morning.

"Doctor, I don't think I should visit Charlie now."

"Why not?"

"I am so overwhelmed with my problems with Kathy."

"In what way?"

"The couple who is supposed to adopt Kathy's baby has just separated. Now I am stuck with all these medical bills. I don't even know if the baby will make it. Kathy is so depressed."

"Don't worry about your problems. I know several couples who would just be thrilled to have a baby. I will take care of it. Kathy's medical bills will also be paid by them. Now that I have figured out the solution to your problem, do you think you can spare an hour for Charlie?"

"Yes, I can. I will be there at 4:30 p.m. today. I will have you paged."

Dr. Olsire went back to the operating room to scrub with the second year resident. The operation went smoothly. After he was finished, Michael went to the social spot to get a cup of coffee.

"Dr. Olsire---Dr. Olsire, Ext. 7118."

"That's the information desk." Dr. Olsire rang ext. 7118.

"Dr. Olsire, I am the receptionist at the information desk. A Mrs. Patty Singleton is waiting for you."

"I will be there shortly."

Dr. Olsire fetched Patty at the information desk. He took her to the room of Charlie Singleton on the sixth floor. Charlie's face gleamed when he saw Patty. Patty was beside herself. She did not know how to act. She didn't know whether she should shake Charlie's hand or hug him. Dr. Olsire broke the ice.

"I will have to leave the two of you so that you can catch up from where you left off."

"How are you, Charlie?"

"I am doing much better, thanks to Dr. Olsire's expert care. How are the twins?"

"They are both fine."

"Did they finish high school?"

"Yes. Michelle is presently working as a secretary. Kathy works at a fast food store."

"When will they visit me?"

"As soon as both of them are able to take a day off. Charlie, you have to tell me where you have been living for the past two years."

"Do you really want to know?"

"Yes, I do."

"I have been living in the streets of center city Philadelphia. Three months after I threw you and the kids out, the house was foreclosed! It went up for Sheriff's Sale two months later.

"Oh, my God!"

"Not only was a street person, but I also became hooked up with a drug dealer and later on started pushing drugs myself to survive."

"I can't believe it."

"It's true. This drug dealer is ruthless. He also uses the disabled to sell drugs. He practically controls the drug trade in downtown Philadelphia."

"How come he is getting away with it?"

"He is a powerhouse."

"How did you get admitted to this hospital?"

"The rescue squad brought me here. I was unconscious when they brought me to the accident ward of this hospital. I had surgery, and, since my admission, Dr. Olsire has been taking care of me. He is a concerned physician. How is your mom?"

"She is doing well. She has been very supportive of us since you threw us out two years ago."

"Please do not remind me of all the heartaches I have caused you. If only I could bring back the past, I would do it."

"We can't dwell on it. We should never look back, but should look forward to the future."

"Do you really mean that?"

"Yes, I do."

"Does that mean I will be able to live with you and the twins when I get discharged?"

"I don't know yet. We would not be able to rent an apartment with what I make. I do not know if Mom will let you stay in her house. You would have to enter a rehabilitation hospital first. Then we can make a decision about our future. Right now, the twins and I do not even have good medical insurance. The place where I work is offering only HMO. I can probably get you on as one of my dependents. Charlie, I must go now."

Patty squeezed Charlie's hand but was hesitant to hug him. Charlie's eyes followed Patty's steps as she walked out of the room.

Patty went directly to Southern Hospital where Kathy was confined. Kathy kissed her mom.

"Mom, you look so haggard. Did you just get off from work?"

"No. I went to the hospital to visit your father."

"What? How come you did not tell us?"

"I did not want Grandmom to know. I don't know how she will take this."

"Did you tell Dad that I am pregnant and not married?"

"No."

"When will you tell him?"

"I don't know yet. I am afraid if I tell him now he would not be able to accept it. He might develop more guilt."

"How about Michelle? Did you tell her that you were going to visit Dad?"

"No. I don't know how I will tell Grandmom either. Please, pray that Grandmom will find it in her heart to forgive your Dad."

"I will."

"Well, tomorrow I am going to get my approval for HMO Healthcare Insurance. You are going to be covered because there is no pre-existing condition requirement."

"Mom, I am so leery about HMO. I have heard so many bad things about it."

"I know, but we have no choice. I would not be able to afford Blue Cross and Blue Shield. It is too expensive!"

"Does Dr. Pore participate in HMO?"

"No, you would have to switch to an HMO doctor. I will be getting a list of HMO participating physicians, and then we both can go over it. We can choose from the list of primary care physicians and obstetricians."

"Mom, I am really scared of a physician from an HMO list. I hear all sorts of horror stories from former HMO patients, and I am just scared. I hope I get lucky and find a physician who is an HMO not by choice, but by economic pressure."

"Let's hope for the best."

Kathy's obstetrician, Dr. Pore, informed her that he just got a call from the HMO office telling him to discharge her.

"I told them I am not discharging you with your condition, and, if HMO wants you to be discharged, HMO will have to sign the discharge papers. That's all there is to it."

"Thank you, Dr. Pore. I wish I could stay under your care."

"I will have to repeat the ultrasound in a couple of days. Then I will make my decision whether to discharge you or not."

Patty Singleton was with Kathy when the Ultrasound was repeated. The placenta did not occupy as much of the mouth of the womb any longer, and there was no evidence of Abruptio Placenta. Dr. Pore rechecked Kathy's blood count. The hemoglobin was 11 grams. He instructed Kathy to stay on bedrest, to take her iron pills with laxative, to take her vitamins, and to eat a well-balanced diet. Patty and Kathy were very thankful for Dr. Pore's kindness and concern.

"Don't forget to get a referral slip from your primary care physician and to give this summary of your hospital care to your HMO obstetrician. If you have any questions about the care I rendered here, please call me. Please let me know how you make out. Good luck."

Patty called several primary care physicians' offices. Most of them had already filled up their patient quota. She finally found one. She went to the primary care physician's office. The office was crowded. Patty had to wait an hour before she was able to see the receptionist to get the referral slip. It was like an assembly line. The receptionist was abrupt and asked a lot of questions as if Patty were trying to steal money from her pocketbook. All of a sudden, a lady screamed in the center of the waiting room.

"I want a referral slip to a neurologist. I have had this headache for six weeks, and you are trying to deny me referral to a specialist! If something happens to me, I will sue you for medical malpractice!"

The secretary was beside herself. She quickly handed the referral slip to the furious patient.

The patient left hurriedly, but she could be heard saying, "These money hungry doctors should be sued. They don't care about patients. All they care about is lining their pocketbooks."

After Patty got the referral slip, she went directly to work. She told her co-workers what had happened at the primary care physician's office.

"HMO is a terrible insurance, but we have no alternative. Dr. Olsire told me that it is illegal for an employer to offer only HMO. The HMO Federal Act of 1973 states that HMO insurance should be offered only as an option."

One of the co-workers said, "I hope I stay healthy so that I will not have to go to HMO doctors."

CHAPTER IV

On June 30, 1983, Carousel Hotel was bustling with activity. It was lavishly decorated with medical motif, including a huge heart behind the presidential table. It was a surprise retirement party for Dr. Jay Simmons. Dr. Simmons had trained physicians all over the world. There were about 600 ex-residents, students, and their wives who responded to the invitations and were expected to attend the grand finale of the brilliant career of this distinguished surgeon, author, writer, lecturer, friend, and mentor. Dr. Simmons was unaware of the party. His daughter, Debbie, and her friends, Drs. Estela and Jorge Cortez, managed to keep this surprise from Dr. Simmons.

All the guests stayed at the Carousel Hotel and other nearby hotels in downtown Philadelphia. Debbie and her friends planned a big catered brunch at the sprawling Bryn Mawr mansion of Dr. Simmons the next day. Even the nuns from the neighboring college were invited to the brunch. Dr. Simmons was the personal physician of this order of nuns. He was also on the board of directors of the college.

The affair started on time at 6:30 p.m. Dr. James Dillon, who was supposed to go back to Trinity College in Ireland, came early to help with the last minute details. Laura Secula and Michael Olsire came next. By seven o'clock, every one of the guests had arrived.

Debbie called from their home. She was supposed to take Estela and Jorge to dinner at the Carousel Hotel. Dr. Simmons was asked to join them.

As soon as the security guard signaled the arrival of the honoree and his party, the lights in the banquet room were turned off. As the honoree entered the door of the banquet room, the band started playing "For He's a Jolly Good Fellow," and the lights were turned on.

Dr. Simmons' face gleamed with mixed surprise and joy. He didn't know what to say. He did not expect this overwhelming display of respect and love from his former students and residents. Dr. Simmons could still remember each and every one of the residents' and students' faces and even some of their names.

The party was for renewing acquaintances and friendships. Every one of the residents was reminiscing about old times. They were talking about their baptism of fire in medical school and residency, their rite of passage.

Each table had three big, red roses as the centerpiece. Each table sat ten people. Table one was the honoree's table. Dr. Simmons sat with his daughter, Debbie, and his son and daughter-in-law and their two daughters.

The menu was fruit cup, filet mignon, mashed potatoes, and green beans almondine, with strawberry shortcake and coffee for dessert.

The sit-down dinner was preceded by cocktails and hors d'oeuvres.

Debbie and Dr. Simmons went around each table to greet everyone, to say thank you for coming half way around the world for the party, and to have pictures taken with the guests at each table.

After dinner, everyone enjoyed dancing to the nostalgic music. People were mingling to meet old acquaintances and friends'.

There was also a skit and roast improvised by each group of former residents. These skits and roasts were all expressions of respect, love, and farewell to a well-respected and loved professor.

Before the night ended, Jorge Cortez delivered a speech on behalf of all the residents. He thanked everyone for coming to honor a very special doctor.

Jorge said, "I don't know how to start and end this speech, but I do know how to sum it up. Thank you, Dr. Simmons, for being such a patient, brilliant, humane, and compassionate physician and for being such a role model for all of us. We are proud to have been taught by you, influenced by you, and we all hope we will always practice medicine the way you taught us: the patient should always be our first priority, and we should always try to put ourselves in the shoes of the patient."

Jorge offered a toast to him, and everyone toasted the incredible physician.

Dr. Simmons, Debbie, Estela, and Jorge were the last ones to leave the hotel. As soon as they got home, Jorge and Dr. Simmons went to sleep. They were both exhausted. Debbie and Estela talked for an hour before they went to sleep.

By 9:00 a.m. the next day, the waiters and waitresses from the catering restaurant were already busy preparing brunch. There were about 60 round tables which sat ten each.

The buffet menu consisted of eggs, beef hash, bacon, pancakes, different kinds of cereals, and fresh fruits.

This time, Dr. Simmons and everyone had a chance to exchange pleasantries, to swim, and to play golf and tennis. The women played cards, and some of them played monopoly.

The party lasted until 3:00 p.m., at which time each and every guest said goodbye. There was also picture taking before everyone left.

Estela and Debbie stayed at the gazebo and reminisced about their internship at Bellevue Hospital in New York. It was through Debbie that Estela had met Jorge three years ago. Debbie had taken Estela with her for a weekend in Philadelphia. Usually, Dr. and Mrs. Simmons invited a couple of residents for dinner on Saturday evening. It was on this particular Saturday that Jorge met Estela.

Jorge did not lose any time. The weekend after their meeting, he went to New York and took Estela and Debbie to a Broadway play. His every other Saturday commuting to New York eventually became a routine and was quite expensive, too.

Finally, after one year of persistence, he gave Estela an engagement ring, and they were married quietly in Philadelphia with Dr. and Mrs. Simmons as sponsors.

CHAPTER V

Estela moved to Philadelphia. She applied for a residency at Philadelphia General Hospital. It was a very hard grind for Estela, juggling her duties as a resident and a housewife. The hours were so ungodly. One and a half years after they were married, Estela became pregnant. This pregnancy was unplanned, so she was quite upset about it. So was Jorge! Estela was quite depressed for several weeks. She was unable to retain any food. She took Bendectin throughout her pregnancy. She was so exhausted during her first few weeks of pregnancy that she collapsed at work.

She took off for one week after she was discharged from the hospital.

Jorge told her, "Estela, I think it's time you quit the residency program. It is getting to be a hassle for you."

"I know some of the male residents were upset when I took off, and they had to fill the slack. I would do the same for them, though, if they became ill."

By the fourth month, Estela felt much better even though she continued to take Bendectin. She ate more nutritious food and took her prenatal vitamins and iron.

"Oh my God, my baby is moving and jumping!" exclaimed Estela. She immediately called Jorge. "I am a mother-to-be! I can feel the baby move around and kick."

"I'm going to bring my stethoscope home so I can listen to the baby's heartbeat."

As soon as Estela got home, she called Debbie in New York.

"I'm feeling great. I can feel the baby kicking."

"I am so happy for you and Jorge. I hope you will make me the godmother."

"Naturally."

Estela and Jorge's Latin American culture influenced their decision to study the "Lamaze Technique" of childbirth. They attended three classes and practiced regularly at home.

In her fifth month, she started having irregular contractions every now and then, especially when she was very tired.

When she was seven and half months, her painless, irregular contractions became more frequent, so much so that she had to quit her residency and be monitored at home. Her fetal monitor was hooked up with a central monitoring service. The nurse in charge read the tracing twice a day. Early in the morning, two weeks before her due date, the fetal tracing showed decreased fetal heartbeat.

"Estela, call the ambulance in your neighborhood and the hospital delivery room. Also, I am going to call your husband so he can in turn call Dr. Kinney. Don't panic!"

"I won't."

"Your husband and obstetrician should be there as soon as you get there."

Estela could hear the ambulance siren as it arrived five minutes later. Minutes later she was in the delivery room of the hospital. Her husband and obstetrician were already waiting in the delivery room.

"Jorge, I'm scared. Something might happen to the baby!"

"Honey, everything will be fine. Dr. Kinney is right here. He is getting ready to do a C-section on you."

"Why?"

"The baby's cord is about to prolapse, but everything is being taken care of. The nurse just instilled saline into your bladder to prevent pressure of the head on the baby's cord."

"Let's take Estela to the Caesarean section room now."

"Jorge, are you going in with me?"

"Yes, of course. I will be there to hold your hand."

"Estela, the anaesthesia department is not here yet. I have to get started immediately because we're racing against time. I will give you local anaesthesia."

"Do whatever you think is best to facilitate the delivery of my baby, doctor."

"I will."

Estela was prepped briskly. The fetal heartbeat was checked again prior to draping.

"Estela, I am now instilling Xylocaine where I will make the incision. Please, bear with the pulling."

Within three minutes, Dr. Kinney was ready to pull out the baby from the uterine incision. The baby cried immediately after suction of the nasopharynx. The baby was handed to the neonatologist.

"What apgar did you give her?"

"I gave her an apgar of eight and nine."

"Thank God, our baby is fine!"

"Dr. Kinney, could you please put me to sleep now?"

"Alright, the anesthesiologist will give you a crash induction."

"Thank you, doctor."

Estela was now asleep. Jorge stayed to watch the closure of the abdominal incision. Finally, the operation was over. Jorge and Dr. Kinney both talked to the nurse in charge of the Fetal Monitoring Service to thank her and compliment her for her diagnostic acumen.

"Miss Stutt, everything went well, and we had a cute baby girl with good apgar. Thanks for your sharp judgement."

"Dr. Kinney, you did a great job. I would not hesitate to refer a friend to you."

"Thank you. I hope you will send us healthy patients."

"Dr. Kinney, I cannot thank you enough for your timely intervention. Estela and I are really very grateful."

"Anytime. I am just glad we got the baby delivered as soon as we did."

"May I stay with Estela until she wakes up?"

"By all means. I will tell the nurse to get you some lunch, too."

Jorge went to the nursery as soon as Estela was wheeled into the recovery room. The baby weighed eight pounds two ounces and the length was 23 inches.

He went back to the recovery room again. He held Estela's hand and tried to wipe the sweat from her face and forehead.

Finally, lunch was served. He did not realize how hungry he was until he finished his meal. He was still hungry.

"I'm going to the snack shop. Please tell Estela in case she wakes up while I'm downstairs. I am also going to call Dr. Simmons and Debbie."

Dr. Kinney got a call from the utilization reviewer of insurance on the third post-operative day of Estela's stay.

"Mrs. Cortez should be discharged today."

"What is your name and specialty? What is your license number? Are you retired or a practicing physician?"

"I am an internist."

"You are not surgically qualified to tell me when I should discharge my patient."

"But I won't pay the hospital."

"I am going to appeal it. You are not acting in the best interest of the patient! And, you call yourself a patient advocate! Do you know who you are and what you are?"

"Yes, I do."

"Well, as far as I'm concerned, you are the advocate of the insurance company and of your pocketbook. You are a medical prostitute."

The physician utilization reviewer hung up on Dr. Kinney.

"Jorge, I just had a run in with the physician utilization reviewer of the insurance company. These people don't care as long as they are paid by the insurance company. They have betrayed the medical profession. I think the Aesculapius should be changed into a dollar sign."

"I know. It's so discouraging. We have lost the freedom to practice good medicine."

"It is mostly the fault of the medical profession. We have failed to police ourselves. Conspiracy of silence is still alive and well. I'm not going to discharge Estela today. As long as I have good documentation, the insurance company just can't deny payment to the hospital."

"Thank you, Dr. Kinney."

"You are welcome."

On the fifth post-op day, Estela was discharged with the baby. Estela took six weeks off and tried to learn as much as she could about baby care and the baby's sleeping and eating habits. There were days when she became frustrated because the baby would cry for hours before she could find out what was going on with her.

There is no such thing as learning everything in baby care. Motherhood is on-the-job training. No matter what the experts say, every baby has different needs and idiosyncracies.

Estela went back to her residency after her six-week postpartum check-up. Every day was a struggle for her just to get up and get the baby ready to go to the babysitter. The babysitter did not live far from her apartment. The middle-aged lady took care of about ten children ranging in age from newborn to five years. She had her hands full.

Estela would notice sometimes that Nedda's butt was red with diaper rash. There were days when she was colicky and cried all the time. But, as a whole, Nedda was doing well until her eighth month, when Estela noticed her irregular bowel movements. One time she did not move her bowels for four days. She was colicky, but she didn't throw up. Estela and Jorge were frustrated. Nedda's constipation and colic went on for three to four months. They had Nedda's stool checked for bacteria and parasites. The stool examination was normal.

One day Estela decided to surprise the babysitter and went to the apartment early to pick up Nedda. As soon as she entered the apartment, she noticed the smell of gas permeating the whole room. The gas stove was on, on low. To her surprise, she found all the children sleeping on the carpet. All of them were dirty. Some of them had left-over food on their bibs. The sitter was nowhere to be found. Estela was very upset. She went to the different rooms of the apartment to look for her. Still, no sign of the babysitter. She checked each of the children to see if they were fine. Each of the children seemed to be okay. She went downstairs to the apartment manager. She found out that the babysitter went to work daily and didn't come back until three-thirty in the afternoon. She called the police. The babysitter was reported to the Department of Health and Human Services. Estela found out that she did not have a babysitting license. Estela called all the parents of the other children and told them what she had discovered.

Estela called Jorge and told him that she was quitting her residency. She would stay home and take care of Nedda.

"I should really be with her. I missed the first time she said Da-Da and Ma-Ma. I missed the first time she crawled, sat, and rolled over. I missed the first time she smiled and cooed, all the special little things."

Nedda celebrated her first birthday. It was quite a big party for a girl her age!

"I invited all the children of my co-residents. I also invited all the kids watched by Susana, the babysitter."

CHAPTER VI

Patty was unable to visit Charlie prior to his discharge to a Germantown boarding home, courtesy of medical assistance. He would have to have his clotting factor checked twice a week for follow-up and to have the dose of Coumadin, his blood thinner, adjusted. A nurse from the home healthcare agency would come to the boarding home to check Charlie every week.

Patty took the boarding home address and telephone number from Dr. Olsire.

"I will try to visit Charlie. Kathy is home now. We are now covered by HMO."

"I am so sorry to hear that. I hope you find a primary care physician who really cares about his patients and not about lining his pocketbook first."

There were about eight people in the boarding home. One of them, Vince, had just been discharged from an acute nursing home facility. The other three boarders had just been transferred from another home whose license had been revoked by the city because of longstanding, uncorrected health violations. The other three had been there for months because they had no one to look after them.

Their everyday existence consisted of three regular meals. On Saturdays, they were taken on a bus trip around the city. A visiting nurse came to the boarding home once a week to check the boarders with medical problems.

Charlie Singleton did not get any cash money at all because of his history of alcoholism and drug addiction. If he needed to buy something, he had to tell the boarding home manager who would then buy him whatever he needed.

Most of the boarders were able to take care of their bathing and dressing needs themselves. The boarding home looked like a dormitory. It had two huge rooms with four beds in each. It had a common kitchen, a common bathroom, and one big living room.

Sometimes, the boarders got so bored that they volunteered to lick stamps and fill the envelopes for a charitable organization.

It had been a month since Charlie moved to the boarding home. He had not touched any alcohol or drugs at all.

His prothrombin level was under control, and Dr. Olsire was very happy about this. Dr. Olsire called him every week to update him on his prothrombin level and to see how he was doing.

Patty Singleton had not called or visited Charlie. Kathy was back in the hospital because of toxemia. She was also having problems with HMO. The HMO utilization reviewer wanted her discharged and followed at home. Well, Patty had learned how to deal with HMO just by sitting in the primary care physician's waiting room. She had learned a lot from the disgruntled and well-informed HMO subscribers. She had had it with HMO. One day, she was so angry that she called the HMO office.

"Please stop calling the hospital about having my daughter discharged. I am going to call the press and television. Better still, I will sue you if something happens to the baby and my daughter. I mean it."

The HMO utilization reviewer backed down. The reviewer called the obstetrician and told him that the patient could stay until delivery.

Charlie became very depressed when Patty did not visit or call him. He became very withdrawn. He usually sat in one corner of the room looking at the ceiling and would not say a word. There were times when he completely and absolutely refused to eat the entire day. His lack of appetite got worse until, three weeks later, the manager noticed something unusual about Charlie.

"Charlie, do you feel alright? Your skin looks yellow."

"Get off my back. I am fine. I feel okay. You are always picking on me. I don't even bother anybody. I just want to be left alone."

On August 15, 1983, Charlie had a cup of oatmeal, one boiled egg, and a glass of orange juice. He said he felt like a million dollar man. The boarding home manager, however, noticed that Charlie's eyes were also getting yellow.

The next day, Charlie could not get out of bed at all. He felt very weak and nauseous. The boarding home manager called Dr. Olsire.

"I will send the hospital ambulance, and I am going to admit Charlie. Did Patty Singleton call or visit him?"

"No."

Dr. Olsire decided to call Patty. Mrs. Collins answered the phone.

"Kathy has been in the hospital for almost a month now with toxemia. She is now about thirty weeks pregnant. Patty had to run to the hospital to sign the permit for Kathy's emergency Caesarean section."

"I hope everything will be fine."

"I hope so, too. Doctor, please call us back. Patty needs to talk to someone whom she can trust."

"I will. I have to run to the accident ward now; the ambulance carrying Charlie just pulled in. I will talk to you later."

Charlie Singleton was a direct admission. Dr. Olsire pulled out all the charts from Charlie's previous admissions. Dr. Olsire did the history and physical examination himself.

"How long ago did you notice changes in the color of your urine or stool?"

"Two weeks ago."

"Have you been drinking recently?"

"No."

"How much weight have you lost since your discharge from the hospital?"

"Twenty pounds."

"When did you lose your appetite?"

"As soon as I got to the boarding home."

"Did you notice yellowing of your skin?"

"Yes, but I tried to deny it."

"How long have you been drinking?"

"Heavy drinking started four years ago, after I lost my job. I drank 18 oz. everyday. It runs in my family. My two brothers and my father were all recovered alcoholics. All of them died later from liver disease. A few months before I threw out Patty and the twins, my mother was diagnosed as having breast cancer. She died on the day my house was foreclosed."

"What a tragic life! How about your wife?"

"My wife never touched alcohol. She is a very strong and disciplined woman. After my house was foreclosed, I was forced to live in the street. Being homeless completely wiped out whatever self-esteem I had. That's why I became an easy victim of this powerful drug dealer. I was forced to panhandle to support my drug addiction. He not only got us hooked and made money on us regularly, but we also became his drug distributors in the streets when we sold crack and cocaine. At midnight, he would visit us. He would bring a long syringe of 50 cc of cocaine and would use the same needle to inject each of us, usually about fifty homeless people. He got blood from each and every one of us before he reused the needle. He had us convinced that this was the only way of really getting high. He also took all the money from our panhandling, and whatever money we earned from selling drugs. He is a monster."

Dr. Olsire just listened and said, "How sad that one person can be so driven by greed to completely ignore the fact that he is destroying people's lives."

In the process of Dr. Olsire's physical examination of Charlie, he noticed the liver to be enlarged and slightly tender. Stat blood count and liver enzyme studies showed anemia and elevated liver enzymes. Charlie was treated conservatively with intravenous fluids, vitamins, and a high protein diet. He was weighed daily to monitor his weight. Once his nausea had disappeared, he started taking oral feedings. The Ultrasound of his abdomen showed the liver to be enlarged. No abnormal echogenic pattern was noted. Fourteen days later, Charlie was sent back to the boarding home.

Patty was unable to visit him. Kathy had a very complicated delivery. She had postpartum hemorrhage and almost died. The baby was only three lbs. and one oz. The baby did not grow inside her womb because of anemia and toxemia. Patty called Charlie prior to his discharge to the boarding home.

"Charlie, I am sorry I could not be there. Kathy is still very sick. She went into heart failure, and the poison from toxemia almost shot her kidneys. Her heart became enlarged. She will have to be on heart medicine, and she will have to be followed up by a cardiologist. I hope Dr. Dough does not give me a hard time when I ask for a referral to take Kathy to a cardiologist."

"Patty, I understand. Kathy needs you right now. Just keep me posted on her progress."

"Take care, Charlie. I will call you in the boarding home."

"Goodbye, Patty."

When Charlie got back to the boarding home, he had to be moved to an improvised room. His fellow boarders teased him because he had to be isolated. Sometimes, nobody talked to him. They were afraid that he would transmit to them whatever infection he had.

Life in the boarding home for him was very lonely. For the first time in his life, he felt isolated and unwanted. Everything he ate or drank was in a plastic container. The boarding home manager would put the food by the door, and he would grab it from behind the door. He had not taken a shower for five days since his discharge. The visiting nurse had given him a sponge bath the day before, but he still looked shabby and sweaty. The high humidity and temperature did not help either. The air conditioning in the boarding home had been broken down for five days.

Patty called Charlie. "Kathy will be discharged by early next week. She will have to choose a cardiologist to follow her cardiac complications. There are no HMO cardiologists in the neighborhood."

"Before you do anything, please ask Dr. Olsire for a good cardiologist."

"I will do that."

Patty called Dr. Olsire.

"How is Kathy doing?"

"She is doing better. Dr. Olsire, could you please give me the name of a good cardiologist?"

"No problem. You can go to Dr. Ceyel. Be sure you get a referral slip from Dr. Dough so you are not stuck with the medical bills."

"I will. Thank you very much."

Kathy was about to be discharged. Her appointment with Dr. Ceyel was on September 1, 1983.

"Please bring your EKG tracing and echocardiogram so that I can compare them with the EKG and echocardiogram which I will be taking on Kathy."

"Yes, doctor. I am going to pick them up on our way to your office."

Ten days before their appointment to see Dr. Ceyel, Patty dropped by the office of Dr. Dough to pick up the referral slip.

Patty said, "Please give me two referral slips so I don't have to go back and forth for our next visit with Dr. Ceyel."

"I can't do that. You might need to see him only once."

"That's not what I was told. Kathy has Idiopathic Cardiomyopathy. This is a very serious complication. She will have to see the cardiologist regularly until the size of her heart becomes normal again."

"Well, you will have to come back every time she has an appointment with the cardiologist."

"You really live up to your name, Dr. Dough."

Two days before she was to be discharged, Kathy became withdrawn. She hardly talked to anyone, even to the nurses who were taking care of her. She could not sleep either. Kathy became very depressed. Patty called Dr. Olsire for advice.

"Patty, I think Kathy is going through postpartum blues or is feeling the pain and guilt of having to give up her baby. You must sit down with her and try to explain to her young mind why she has to give up the baby for adoption."

Patty went back to the hospital and tried to reason with Kathy.

"This is the best thing for you and the baby."

"But, Mom, I love my baby. I don't want to give him up. I want to take care of him."

"I know that. I love my grandson, too. I am trying to do what is best for all of us. Who is going to take care of him when I go to work and you go to school? Grandmom can't do it. She can hardly walk with her arthritis, much less take care of a baby. Michelle can't babysit either. She has to work and go to night school at the same time. Don't worry; Dr. Olsire assured me that this couple will really take good care of the baby. They are also in a position to give this baby the best upbringing and education. We must trust Dr. Olsire's judgement and concern for all of us."

Before Kathy was finally discharged on Aug. 25, 1983, she formally relinquished her parental rights. Patty took off for one week just to take care of her. The baby stayed in the hospital nursery. The baby's weight was only three pounds one ounce on Kathy's discharge.

The adopting parents sent a big basket of fruit to Patty's house signed: With Love and Concern, The Adopting Parents. The short note read:

Dear Kathy,

Thank you for your precious little gift to us, the Gift of Life. We will never forget you in our prayers. Baby Geoffrey will surely be nurtured with love, kindness, and compassion. You have made us the happiest couple on earth. You have indeed made the greatest and ultimate sacrifice by giving of yourself, little Geoffrey.

God Bless!

Your Friends,
Geoffrey's other Mom
and Dad

After Kathy and Patty read the card with the short note, they both broke down.

"Dr. Olsire was right in choosing this couple. They seem like caring and loving people. We have to pray that they will always think of Geoffrey this way."

On Sept. 11, 1983, Kathy had her first visit with the cardiologist. Dr. Ceyel was very pleasant and explained everything to Patty and Kathy. He continued Kathy's medication,

Capoten. He also repeated the EKG and the echocardiogram. He asked Kathy if she had had influenza during her pregnancy.

"No, the only complications I had were the bleeding and toxemia."

"Your heart size is not what I would like it to be. But the size has decreased a little bit. I would like to check you again in two months. In the meantime, continue your iron, vitamins, and Capoten."

CHAPTER VII

Laura Secula and Michael Olsire had become good friends. They had so much in common. Both were aspiring surgeons and were training in university hospitals. Dr. Olsire was a first year fellow while Laura was in her third year of residency. They shared the same ideas and priorities when it came to taking care of patients.

They both shared a fondness for the arts. Everytime there was a new play in town, they always found time to see it.

When they were off, they were usually jogging or walking around the Art Museum. For them, walking and jogging were the best ways to ward off the stresses of surgical training.

One morning while jogging, they got into a big discussion about healthcare and how politicians had messed up the healthcare system.

"I am so disgusted with what's going on with healthcare. We can't even make our own decisions on how to treat patients. The doctors and nurses who work for the utilization review companies don't realize that they could be legally liable if the patient dies or suffers when discharged prematurely."

"So, what should we do then?"

"We have to educate the medical students, the patients, and the public."

"Where do we start?"

"Well, let's start with the Medicare mess and the DRG. The DRG is not saving money at all. Money that should be spent on patient care is being spent on administrative cost and paper work. It's also draining the nursing profession. The burnout rate of nurses is high. It's too stressful to work in hospitals nowadays. The elderly are admitted too sick and are discharged prematurely."

"It's a shame."

"We should also educate the public about how the government spent 369 million dollars of taxpayer money to get the HMO started. I don't know why the government passed this law giving financial incentive to primary care physicians (gatekeepers) to control cost. Actually, this is really a kickback to deny care, hospitalization, and referral to a specialist. The government also protects the HMO's by suing doctors who try to educate the public about the evils of HMO's for antitrust."

"Hippocrates not only must be rolling over in his grave, but probably is doing somersaults as well."

"I know."

"At least I have few more years before I finish my residency."

"Everytime I think that in one year I will be out in practice, I shiver."

"I feel so sad whenever I think of what's in store for all future physicians: litigation, interference from third party payers, government and consumer demands."

"It might be more satisfying just to work in the Indian Reservation. Indian people would be happy and grateful just to have a doctor around. Or, we could apply to Project Hope or Medico."

"We would not have to worry about liability insurance premiums, HMO's, utilization reviewers, DRG, and the peer review organizations."

"I know."

"It is really so unfair."

"The public is successfully being kept in the dark about what is actually going on in the healthcare crisis by the media and the government."

"Healthcare consumers do not realize that the government, employers, commercial insurance companies, and HMO's are rationing care."

"So are the hospitals."

"In what way?"

"When the hospital pharmacy substitutes a less expensive drug or a generic drug for a brand name one without the consent of the ordering physician or of the patient, then this constitutes rationing of healthcare. This could be fraudulent if, when the patient is billed, the bill does not reflect the type of drug given."

"I think this is terrible."

"So do I. Even the gatekeepers from HMO's ration healthcare by ordering less testing, less referral to specialists, and less admissions in order to make more money."

"I don't think it is only rationing. I find it unconscionable that a doctor would treat a patient this way."

"Laura, where have you been? This has been going on since 1977, even though that entity we all call conscience should have long ago stopped the medical profession from being so apathetic to the plight of its patients."

"This is really an abuse of the trust that is placed in a physician. It is a betrayal of the patient's confidence. It is against the Hippocratic Oath."

"Part of this problem is an economic factor. Physicians with debts and just coming out of their residency are the easiest targets."

Michael suddenly changed the subject.

"I am going to come to your hospital after dinner. I will page you when I get there."

"Okay."

It was already seven o'clock when Michael arrived at Northend Hospital. He had Laura paged.

Laura was scrubbed in the O.R. for an emergency appendectomy. She did not get finished until 8:00 p.m. After she was finished talking to the family and explaining to them about the surgical findings, she went up to the social spot, carrying the dinner she had brought from home. Michael was not in the social spot. She went to the information desk.

Michael had fallen asleep on the sofa in front of the information desk.

"Michael, please wake up."

"What time is it?"

"Eight-thirty. I just finished operating on a young kid. He had a ruptured appendix with periappendical abscess. He has been going to his HMO doctor for one week. He treated him for a urinary tract infection. He ordered a blood count and urinalysis, but it took too long to get the laboratory results. Finally, the family brought the kid to the accident ward. He was so dehydrated and toxic. I started him on massive antibiotics."

"When will some of these HMO doctors start thinking of the patient first instead of their bonuses? Doesn't the patient count anymore?"

"I don't know. I am so disillusioned myself. Wait till you hear this one. The patient's mother was telling me that her niece had been complaining of headaches for several weeks. She went to her HMO doctor and asked for a referral slip to go to a neurologist and to have a CAT Scan test. The HMO doctor did not give her a referral slip. He told her that it was emotional stress and that it was all in her head. It was really in her head! She has a brain tumor."

"This type of doctor should be sued. You know, I don't believe in suing people, but, my God, this doctor deserves it! If he does not care about the patient, at least he should be afraid of litigation. But, the way things are, greed is more powerful than the fear of being sued."

"The HMO Federal Act of 1973 should be repealed. The financial incentives should be stopped."

"I guess many young doctors are so overburdened with school tuition bills that they have no choice."

"You always have a choice. Let's eat now before this ravioli gets cold."

"This ravioli really tastes good. Did your Mom make this?"

"Yes, she did. I don't have time to cook. By the time I get home, I am ready to fall asleep. The O.R. schedule has been so hectic lately because most of the patients have come back from the shore. I will be scrubbed the whole day tomorrow."

"I am going to go now. I have to scrub with the first year residents tomorrow. I will make rounds at 6:00 a.m. I will just go back to the hospital. I will call you tomorrow. Good night."

"Michael, I hope you are not busy tonight."

"I hope so, too."

The next morning, Michael called Laura.

"Do you want to see a play tonight?"

"I can't."

"Why not?"

"I have to take Mom to the doctor at seven tonight."

"How about tomorrow?"

"I can't. I have to take Mom to the mall and to the grocery store."

"How about Friday?"

"Friday, I will be on call again."

"Well, I will be talking to you tomorrow. Be sure you write something about the healthcare crisis and send it to your politician, okay?"

"Yes, I will try to write as much as I can."

After work the next day, Laura rushed home. She did not finish in the operating room until 6:00 p.m. She had to recheck the first patient she had operated on that morning. She went to the surgical floor. The young boy who was operated on for a ruptured appendix was doing well.

Laura was finally on her way home. The traffic on Roosevelt Blvd. was at a standstill. There was a big accident near Southampton Road. It took her thirty minutes to get home.

As soon as she drove into their driveway, she saw her mother looking through the window. She rushed upstairs and kissed her mom.

"Mom, I am sorry I am a little bit late."

"Let's go. I don't want to be late for my appointment."

"Don't worry, Mom, we will make it on time."

By the time Laura and Mrs. Secula arrived at the doctor's office, the office was already crowded. Some patients were standing outside the waiting room. Laura noticed HMO posters all over the walls of the doctor's waiting room. There were about twenty patients ahead of them. Laura noticed that they were only paying two dollars.

They waited for two and a half hours before her mother was seen. Laura wanted to talk to the doctor about her mother's medical condition. The doctor said he did not have time to talk to Laura because he was so far behind in his schedule. Laura just bit her tongue. She resented the overscheduling of patients. She told his secretary that she would prefer that her mother be billed.

The secretary said, "We do not bill patients. I want the money now."

Laura gave the secretary a dirty look and said, "Actually, your office owes me and my mother two and half hours of our time. I will send you our bills. Our time is as important as the doctor's time."

The secretary was dumbfounded, but she retorted, "I will relay your message to the doctor."

"Do that please."

On their way home, Laura said to her mom, "I wish you would switch to another doctor who is not HMO."

"But I have been going to him for years."

"I know, but they are overscheduling patients. It's like an assembly line. You are treated just like a number."

"I will think about it."

"Mom, let me write your doctor a letter. I don't want you to pay the bill. I will explain to him why he owes us money."

"Whatever you say, Laura."

As soon as they got home, Laura got a bite to eat. She went upstairs to her room and started writing this letter.

Dear Dr. Dollar:

Please be advised that you owe me and my mother fifty dollars for our time spent waiting in your office.

If you don't realize by now why you owe us money, I'll tell you. As a result of your overscheduling of patients in the office, we had to wait two and a half hours before my mother was seen.

Moreover, the HMO patients were paying only two dollars. Are you trying to make my mother subsidize those two-dollar office visits?

A response to this letter will be greatly appreciated and is expected.

Sincerely,

Laura Secula

Dr. Dollar was furious when he got the letter from Laura. He called her in the hospital. "This is Dr. Dollar. Dr. Secula, you can take your mother to another doctor if you are not satisfied with my care."

"That's what I am planning to do. I find it insensitive to patients that you would make them wait two and a half hours in your office. I think you are overscheduling your patients. The patient's time is as important as your time."

"I don't need a lecture from you. You don't know how hard it is to be a practicing physician nowadays. We are under a lot of pressure from everyone."

"So am I. I know what is going on, but you don't take it out on the victims, the patients. The patients don't even have an idea of what's going on. I'm glad I am able to provoke your anger. I hope you do something about the situation. Thank you for your time."

Laura went up to the surgical floor to make rounds on post-operative patients. Then she proceeded to the operating room.

Code 1, Room 6 O.R. === Code 1, Room 6 O.R. === Code 1, Room 6 O.R.

Everyone ran to room six. All the people in the O.R. were busy trying to resuscitate a man who suddenly had developed a 106° temperature and rigidity. By the time Laura got to room six, the patient was already dead.

"My God, this day is a downer and it's only Monday."

Laura called Michael in the afternoon.

"We had an anaesthetic death."

"What caused it?"

"Malignant hyperthermia. It was terrible. I could sympathize with both the family and the anesthesiologist. It was a scary situation. The patient's temperature went up to 106°. Then the patient became rigid. All the efforts to save him failed."

"I'd hate to be in the shoes of the surgeon. How did the family take it?"

"The wife was admitted to the Coronary Care Unit. She developed severe chest pains and passed out after she was told about what had transpired in operating room. I hope she has no myocardial infarction."

"I hope so, too! I have bad news for you as well. Charlie Singleton just called me. He's had a cough since his discharge. I am waiting for him now. I have to do a chest X-Ray and HIV test."

CHAPTER VIII

On November 12, 1983, Charlie's HIV test came back positive. The Western blot was also positive, and he had developed pneumocystic Carinii Pneumonia. He was started on AZT and Pentamidine in the hospital. His T-cell count was less than 250 per cubic mm. of blood.

On further questioning, Dr. Olsire found out that Charlie had had a dry cough, sweats, and severe diarrhea for two weeks after his discharge.

"Charlie, why didn't you call me sooner with all the symptoms you have been having?"

"I was attributing most of my symptoms to the poor air conditioning of the boarding home."

"Charlie, I have started you on two experimental medications, AZT and Pentamidine. The AZT is for your positive HIV and Pentamidine is for your pneumonia. As soon as you get situated, please call Patty."

"I don't know what to say. I have given them too much heartache already. Kathy is not even well yet. Her heart has not gone down to its normal size."

"But, I think she should know about your medical condition."

"I have to think about it."

"How about calling her in two days?"

"It's a deal."

"I will see you tomorrow."

"Please, say hello for me to your friend, Dr. Laura."

"Will do."

Michael called Laura. "I have bad news for you. Charlie Singleton was just admitted with full blown AIDS. I am scared. I have to get tested for AIDS, too."

"I understand what you mean. But, I think Charlie developed the AIDS from drug abuse and not from multiple blood transfusions."

"I understand that, but I got stuck with the surgical knife accidentally while I was operating on Charlie. God, please give me a break."

"Michael, calm down. I am sure your immune system is better than Charlie's. I am with you. I pray that you do not get infected because of that accident."

"I hope so. Thank you for your pep talk."

Michael went to the chief pathologist and requested that he be tested for AIDS. The result would not be in until two weeks later.

Michael went back to the fourth floor to talk to Charlie.

"Charlie, were you able to eat your lunch?"

"Yes, I tried very hard even though I didn't feel like eating. I would like to see Kathy's baby boy."

"I don't think that will be possible."

"Why not?"

"The baby was taken by the adopting parents five days after Kathy was discharged."

"Do you have any idea who adopted the baby?"

"I am not in a position to tell you. I am sorry."

"That's alright. I will call Patty tomorrow."

"Do that."

Charlie called Patty at home. Patty was quite surprised and upset to find out that Charlie was back in the hospital.

"What's wrong, Charlie?"

"Patty, brace yourself and don't get upset with what I have to tell you."

"What's wrong with you?"

"I have developed a deadly disease through my own fault. I have AIDS!"

"What?!"

"I have AIDS, an immune deficiency disease."

"Oh my God! This is terrible. What have you done to yourself?"

"Well, I am to blame for all my problems. I became a drug addict and a drug peddler while I was living in the streets. It's a long story. The homeless people around the Grand Old Hotel are victims of a legal powerhouse. We were blackmailed into doing this illegal drug peddling. We were left no other choice. Please, don't tell Kathy and Michelle. I will have to tell them myself when you come to visit me."

"That's your decision. I have to respect it."

After Patty hung up, she became hysterical. "Dear God, help us and give us strength and courage to deal with our problems."

Mrs. Collins heard Patty crying.

"What's wrong, Patty?"

"Charlie has AIDS."

"Do the kids know?"

"Not yet. I can't tell them until I talk to Dr. Olsire. I tried to call Dr. Olsire before Charlie called, but he was operating. I left a message for him. I am going to call him again as soon as I have put myself together. I hope he levels with me."

"I hope so. Patty, get some sleep. You look so tired. All this worry about Kathy and Charlie is really running you down."

"I know."

Late in the afternoon, Dr. Olsire called Patty.

"Dr. Olsire, thank you for returning my call. How is Charlie? How serious is his condition? I know AIDS is a very fatal disease. How long is he going to live?"

"I don't know. It is really hard to tell. He has lost twenty pounds since his discharge four weeks ago. He also has pneumonia. He has the full-blown manifestations of AIDS. I would guess probably three to six months. I hate to do this, though, because, when I do this, I feel as if I am giving a death sentence to a patient."

"I understand."

"The best thing for you and your girls to do is to visit Charlie regularly. Make him feel needed and show him that you care. I am sure he would appreciate whatever caring you show him."

"We will."

Patty called Michelle at work. "Your father is back in the hospital. Please come home early so that we can all visit him. He is in serious condition."

"What's wrong?"

"I can't tell you."

"I will be home by five o'clock." "Kathy and I will be ready by then." "Is Grandmom coming?"

"I don't think so."

"Let's ask her."

"Alright."

As soon as Michelle got home, Patty and Kathy were already dressed.

"Is Grandmom coming?"

"No. What can I say?"

"Let's go."

On the way to the hospital, they discussed how Kathy and Michelle would approach their father. This would be the first time they saw him since they left their house. It would be their reunion.

Dr. Olsire was waiting for them at the information desk. Dr. Olsire greeted everyone. They proceeded to the fourth floor of the Medical Building. Charlie was sleeping. But, when he heard the footsteps, he awakened. Patty, Kathy, and Michelle kissed and embraced Charlie. Charlie's eyes were gleaming with happiness. Then he started crying and said, "I am sorry for all the heartaches I have caused all of you. I wish I could make up for all the insensitivity and irresponsibility. But, there isn't much time left for me. I can feel my body getting weaker everyday. I don't sleep well because of my hacking cough. My body is starting to dwindle. Every bite of food I take I can hardly chew. I don't even retain it because of my diarrhea. With whatever time I have left, I want to make it up to all of you."

Patty, Kathy, and Michelle started crying. In unison, they all exclaimed, "Please don't talk like that."

Kathy and Michelle both said, "We will visit you, and we also would like to renew our relationship with you. The past has been buried and forgotten."

"Thank you, Dr. Olsire," said Charlie.

"That's alright. I have to finish making my rounds before I visit Laura tonight."

As soon as Dr. Olsire finished making rounds, he called Laura.

"Laura, I would like to drop by your house tonight."

"Okay. Mom cooked a big dinner for us. Come early and have dinner with us."

"Thank you, I will do that."

Michael took Roosevelt Blvd. to get to Laura's house. There was a five-car chain reaction accident at Southampton Rd. Michael was delayed for about thirty minutes before Southampton Rd. was cleared by the police. When he arrived at 90064 Kalina St., he noticed that the house was well-lighted and crowded with people. He knocked at the door. Laura opened it.

"Is there a party going on?"

"Yes, it is Mom's birthday."

"You should have told me. I am so embarrassed. I don't even have a present to give her."

"She is just happy you could come tonight."

"Happy Birthday, Mrs. Secula."

"Michael, I am glad you were able to come."

After all the guests were gone, Michael stayed for a while and talked to Laura, Mrs. Secula, and Jeanie, Laura's younger sister.

"Michael, do you have any relatives in Philadelphia?"

"No, Mrs. Secula. I come from Indiana."

"How about your parents?"

"They both died in a car accident when I was twelve."

"I am sorry to hear that."

"My uncle, a priest, raised me. I grew up in his parish. After graduating from high school, I was able to get a scholarship to Notre Dame, and I worked during the summer to save money to supplement my medical school loan."

"I see. You must have been an altar boy, too."

"I was and I also delivered newspapers everyday to earn extra money."

"Your parents would be so proud of you, if they were here."

"I know. When I think about them, I feel like crying. They died very young at the prime of their lives because of a drunken driver. I am an only child, but I am not spoiled. My uncle always lectured me about honesty, hard work, and fair play. He was so delighted when I told him I wanted to become a doctor. He is very proud of me."

"I can imagine. Well, we will leave so that the two of you can talk."

"Thank you, Mrs. Secula."

"Good night."

"Laura, my test will be back in one week. If my test comes back negative, I would like us to get married."

"But we have only known each other for less than a year!"

"We both know who we are. We are so alike. I know everything will work out for us."

"But I still have one and a half years to finish my residency. You know how stressful it is to be in training and to be married at the same time."

"I understand, but we will be helping each other. I have only one year left and I'll be finishing my fellowship. I could either be a full-time faculty member at the university or go into private practice. In the meantime, you can continue your residency. I will also help with the housework."

"I know that."

"We have to talk about this again. I don't want you to feel pressured."

"I have to think about this seriously. This is a major decision. This is so sudden."

"I will give you two weeks."

"Is that an ultimatum or a threat?"

"It's neither. I am getting too old. I will be thirty-three in one month. I want to see my kids grow up before I get too old. You must understand that you were the first girl I dated seriously. When I was growing up, I didn't have time to date. I was always working or in the library reading about Shakespeare, Longfellow, and Edgar Allan Poe. I love to read these authors' works."

"So do I. I was always working to save money to go to medical school. I started working at age 17. I used to work at a deli and a pharmacy. My father retired early from the police force because of his heart ailment. His first heart attack was at age 46. He had to be reassigned to a desk job on the police force after he recovered. Three years ago, he had a quadruple bypass after his last heart attack. He didn't really feel well after his bypass surgery. He did not try to help himself. It was really a very difficult time for us, especially for Mom. Dad just didn't bounce back to his old self. He missed his work. But the authorities put him on total disability. That really did him in. He didn't have a hobby. After he read the newspaper in the morning, he couldn't really do anything else. There were times that I thought he would drive Mom crazy. But Mom is not a complainer. She took everything in stride. Dad was her whole world. Her life revolved around us. She is a very good mother. I could not ask for a better mom. Jeanie and I are so blessed. I can't just tell Mom I am getting married. She is still mourning Dad's death. The best thing for you to do is to come here more often so that Mom will get used to you."

"I understand what you mean. I will just have to do that."

"I will be talking to you tomorrow."

Before Laura turned off the lights, she watched Michael drive away. She did not realize that her mother was watching her.

"Laura, I think you are in love with Michael."

"I am, but I also want to finish my residency."

"Why? Did Michael ask you to marry him?"

"Yes, but it is happening too fast. I have only known him for less than a year."

"Why, when does he want to get married?"

"As soon as possible. He only has one year left with his fellowship. But I have one and a half years left. It is going to be stressful for both of us."

"Do you love him?"

"Yes, I do."

"Trust yourself and your instincts."

"I will."

The next day, Michael called Laura.

"Thank you for a very lovely evening. But I have another bit of bad news for you."

"What is it?"

"Charlie's two fellow homeless were just admitted last night with ulcers all over their lower extremities. I am waiting for the HIV test results. The medical resident who admitted them told me that they used to share the needle with Charlie."

"That does not prove anything. You don't know how long these guys have been shooting drugs. You don't know how long they have been living in the streets."

"You are right. I should not worry then."

"Please don't worry so much! You are putting yourself under unnecessary pressure."

"I know I should stop worrying. What will be, will be."

Charlie's condition was rapidly deteriorating. His T-cell count did not improve even with high doses of AZT. The lesion in his lungs did not improve either after three weeks of Pentamidine.

"Dr. Olsire, how long do you think it will take for me to improve?"

"I don't know."

"I really appreciate your visits everyday even though you are no longer taking care of me. It is so nice of you to take a personal interest in my medical problem and I can't thank you enough for that. Your girlfriend, Dr. Secula, is a very lucky girl."

"I hope she thinks that way about me, too. It is quite hard for me to distinguish her feelings because she is just a nice person. Sometimes, I don't know if she is just nice to me because I showed concern when her father died in this hospital. I really don't know where I stand with her. I do know we have been friends for less than a year."

"I wish I could see her and tell her myself what kind of a doctor you are."

On Nov. 10, 1983, Michael received a copy of his HIV testing. It was negative. He immediately called Laura, but she was tied up in the operating room. She didn't call back until five o'clock.

"Laura, I have good news for you. My HIV testing and Western Blot were both negative."

"Good, this calls for a celebration then. Why don't you come down to our house for dinner?"

"I would love to."

"Mom would be happy to have you for dinner. She thinks the world of you. We will be waiting for you then. How about coming at seven?"

"I will be there at seven o'clock."

Michael was so excited and happy, not only because his HIV and Western blot tests were negative, but because he could just feel that Laura was as happy as he was about the negative results.

Michael arrived at Laura's house at exactly 7:00 p.m.

Mrs. Secula was busy in the kitchen so Laura gave him some olives to nibble on and a glass of wine.

"I can't drink too much wine. I have to be alert. The patient that we operated on today is not doing well at all. I have my beeper on in case I get called."

"I hope you don't get called. It would really upset Mom. She cooked her specialty just for you."

Dinner was lively. Michael felt very comfortable with Laura's family. This was not the first time that he had eaten in their home. But, somehow, he could sense that the atmosphere was different.

Mrs. Secula broke the ice.

"How many years do you have to finish your fellowship?"

"One year."

"Do you plan to go back to Indiana?"

"I don't think so. I would like to teach for a few years after my fellowship. After that, I would like to start a private practice. It is very hard to start a private practice unless one joins an established group practice. Medical liability insurance costs a lot of money. It is terrible. Even those states who have had tort reform are not doing well either. Something has to be done. Many uninsured people are not getting medical care because of the adversarial relationship between doctors and patients."

"I think the government should get out of the healthcare business. Society also should do something about it. It's not only the fault of the doctors, although I think organized medicine should take responsibility for disciplining its members."

"I could not agree more. There are so many unsung heroes in medicine. But they are all being lumped together with the greedy ones in our profession. It's a shame."

"I know. When I think of what is waiting for me after my residency, it gives me second thoughts on why I became a doctor."

"It's the government's fault, too. Just look at all these lousy healthcare laws that were passed in Congress: the Medicare DRG, the HMO Federal Act of 1973, the Mandatory Generic Drug Substitution. The government has also selectively discriminated against hospitals and physicians in order to cut the federal deficit."

"It's so scary to be a senior citizen. The money that should be spent on healthcare is being spent on paperwork. Typical bureaucracy."

"What can we do about all these problems?" asked Mrs. Secula.

"We have to write our politicians."

"But the politicians are out of touch with reality. They don't use the same hospitals we use. They have Bethesda Hospital at their disposal and at the taxpayer's expense."

"Something has to give. I am quickly approaching the Medicare age."

"We don't have to go far to see the inequity of our healthcare system. For example, Philadelphia has six medical schools, but no city hospital. The poor and uninsured that should have been taken care of by a city hospital cannot get medical care. Either they don't qualify for Medicaid because their salaries are above the poverty guideline set up by the state, or they make money but not enough to pay for private healthcare insurance."

"This is terrible."

"The government should do something about the situation. It should also regulate lawyers and insurance companies. Frivolous medical malpractice suits should be stopped."

"Now that the government has passed the law that would monitor physicians, Congress should enact laws to monitor lawyers and insurance companies as well."

"I could not agree more. But I don't think that will ever happen. Why would lawyers in Congress legislate against themselves? It is very naive of someone to think that Congress would even attempt to pass laws regulating lawyers and insurance companies. These two industries have a very powerful lobby in Congress."

"What's for dessert, Mom?"

"Chocolate Mousse."

"I will just have coffee."

"Why?"

"I am allergic to chocolate."

"Would you care for some more wine?"

"No, thank you. I have to get back to the hospital to see how that patient I operated on today is doing. Mrs. Secula, thank you for a lovely dinner."

"You are welcome."

Laura followed Michael to the door. Their eyes met, and Laura looked down, quite embarrassed. Michael squeezed Laura's hand and smiled. He could see that Laura's face was glowing with a beatific smile. He hesitated to give her a good night kiss. He was afraid Laura would get more embarrassed and upset. Michael was singing while driving. He was sure that Laura was also in love with him. That look in her eyes really betrayed her feelings for Michael.

Michael was talking to himself.

"I will just buy her an engagement ring and pop the question. I will not give her a chance to say no."

CHAPTER IX

Charlie Singleton's condition continued to deteriorate. His mental attitude greatly changed from optimism to pessimism. He developed a tunnelling ulcer in his right leg which gradually affected his walking. It was very painful. He lay in bed most of the time. His medical doctor cautioned him about exercising his legs because of his poor medical history.

"Charlie, please try to prop up your legs. I don't want you to have any more complications in addition to your present condition."

"I understand, Dr. Wittle, but I don't think there is any hope for me. I think it is just a matter of weeks and I will be gone. I feel very badly that I did not even have a chance to see my grandson. Even Dr. Olsire could not help me with the adopting parents."

"Knowing Michael very well, I am sure he tried everything to convince the adopting parents to let you see your grandson. I will talk to Michael about this."

"Thank you, Dr. Wittle. All of you doctors have been wonderful to me. I don't know how I can ever repay all of you."

"Not at all."

Dr. Wittle paged Michael Olsire.

"Michael, I think you should talk to the adopting parents about making arrangements for Charlie Singleton to see the baby before he dies. I don't think he will last that long. AZT and Pentamidine have not helped at all. I think what is keeping him going is his reconciliation with his wife and daughters."

"Tom, I will try to talk again to the adopting parents. I have already asked them a couple of times. I will try my best."

"Please do."

Michael Olsire called his friend.

"Michael, I understand whatever you want to do to help Mr. Singleton have peace with himself. I have to talk with my wife about this matter."

"I will wait for your call."

The next day, Michael was paged by his friend.

"There should be no other people in the room except Charlie, you, and us."

"That's a deal. I will make sure that Patty and the girls are not around when you come with the baby. You will have to come during the day then."

"No problem."

The next morning around nine o'clock, Michael and the adopting parents walked into Charlie's room.

"Charlie, here's your grandson."

Charlie's face brightened up and he looked happy and bewildered. He held the baby's hand. "May I kiss him?"

Michael nodded.

"Thank you for letting me see my grandson. Dr. Olsire, you have been so good to me since the first day I set my foot in this hospital."

Charlie started sobbing. "If only I hadn't become an alcoholic, things would have been different. But it is too late now. I know I only have several weeks to live. I have to make up with my family. Up to now, my mother-in-law has not forgiven me. I wish she would before I face my maker."

"Don't worry, Charlie. I will talk to Mrs. Collins. I have had several conversations with her in the past. I am sure she will weigh whatever I have to tell her."

"I hope so."

Michael and the adopting parents were getting ready to leave when Charlie exclaimed, "May I hold the baby once more?"

Charlie was in tears as he watched them leave the room. Then, he went back to sleep.

Patty and the two girls arrived in the afternoon. They were taken aback when they saw Charlie's face. He looked so happy. The pain in his legs did not even bother him. His reunion with his grandson was a sort of healing for him. It lifted his spirits to new heights. He even felt a little better. Seeing the baby was a turning point in his battle with AIDS.

"Charlie, you look happier and better today," said Patty.

"I am. I had a long talk with Dr. Olsire today. Dr. Olsire is so good to me. He always goes out of his way to help me out. He is one in a million."

"I know. If it had not been for him, we would have been lost trying to get medical attention."

"How is your heart, Kathy? Have you been to the doctor lately?"

"We were in his office today. He wants to see Kathy in four weeks. She is still on medications. We have to make an appointment with Dr. Dough to get a referral slip. I hope he does not give us a hard time. I wish he would give us several referral slips, so that we wouldn't have to go back and forth everytime Kathy needs testing and follow-up. According to Dr. Olsire, we are now stuck with HMO unless I find another job, and the contract includes pre-existing condition clause; otherwise, I will have to take another insurance, but then I would have to wait one year before Kathy would be covered. At the same time, I would have to keep my HMO coverage. There is just no way I can afford to pay two medical insurances."

"I know."

"We just have to leave everything in the hands of God."

"Patty, I had a long talk with Dr. Olsire about your mom. I wish I could make peace with her before I die. I know I sound morbid, but we all know how deadly my disease is. I wish you could talk to her about me."

"Charlie, I have tried many times to talk to her about your illness and your feud, but my mother is quite stubborn. There is nothing more I can do. Kathy and Michelle have tried to talk to her, too. Let's just leave things as they are now. Probably, later on, she will relent."

"I hope so."

"Michelle was able to get a grant. She will be going to Penn State in September. She will take nursing at the Ogontz Campus."

"Dad, I did well on the entrance examination. As soon as I start my clinical subjects, I will be able to work as a nurse's aide at least three days a week. Whatever money I make will be used for my books and allowance."

"That's very thoughtful of you."

"Kathy is going to college, too, as soon as her heart complication reverts to normal."

"I am so proud of my girls. I wish you could be proud of me, too," sobbed Charlie. "I wish things were different."

"Charlie, let us look at the future. Don't dwell on the past. We have to make use of the precious time that God has allotted us. Everything happens for a reason. God does not give us sufferings that we cannot handle."

"You are right, Patty. You have been so good to me and the girls, too."

"Do you want anything special to eat? We can bring you some food from home."

"Thank you, but I don't have that much appetite. Dr. Wittle ordered some Ensure Plus for me. It has given me some strength. The yellow-colored intravenous fluid is vitamins. Dr. Wittle said that I did not lose weight yesterday."

"That's good."

"Dad, we have to go now. It's getting late. Our neighborhood is getting run down by drug abusers. There are so many cars being stolen, and they are not being recovered."

Patty and the girls hugged Charlie. Charlie was misty-eyed while he watched his wife and daughters leave. He said to himself, "If only things were different." He stood by the window and watched them drive away.

As soon as he got into his bed, he turned on the television. He could not believe what he saw! The guy who used to make them sell drugs was giving a press conference about medical malpractice.

"My God, he must be a real shark!"

Charlie immediately dialed the hospital telephone operator.

"Please page Dr. Olsire."

"Dr. Olsire has left. He is off today."

"Thank you. What a lost opportunity!"

The next day, Dr. Olsire visited Charlie.

"I was looking for you yesterday, Doc."

"Why?"

"The guy who used to make us sell drugs was on television."

"What's his name?"

"Robert Smith."

Dr. Olsire went out to the nurses' station and got a yellow page directory. He checked the pages under lawyers.

"Charlie, there are about twenty lawyers here whose name is Robert Smith!"

"I know. Maybe we can call the television station and ask about this guy."

"I don't know if we can do that."

"Do you think you can buy the video?"

"I don't know. It would probably cost an arm and a leg. I could not afford it. But we can always try. So, how is your family?"

"They were here last night. I did not tell them that I saw the baby. I did not want to upset Kathy. She is not well yet. Her heart is still enlarged."

"Kathy has a very, very rare complication. It will take time before her heart goes back to normal size. Let's just hope for the best. What are Dr. Wittle's plans for you?"

"Well, he is giving me my medications, some intravenous vitamins, and Ensure Plus. I feel a bit stronger today. My legs don't hurt as much. I cannot thank you enough for bringing the adopting parents and the baby to see me. It really made me very happy to know that the baby is in good hands. I owe you so much. Can I ask you one more favor, doctor?"

"Sure, Charlie."

"I have three envelopes for you; one is for Patty, the other two are for you. Please don't open yours until I've been gone for two years. Also, would you give Patty her envelope after I'm dead?"

"Don't worry about it, Charlie. I will take care of it. I have to go and see my patients before I leave. I am going to have dinner with Laura and her family."

"Dr. Olsire, Dr. Laura seems really nice and cute, too."

"I know. She is special."

"Please say hello to her for me."
"I will. Get a good night's sleep, Charlie."

CHAPTER X

Michael Olsire was a little bit late because of the heavy traffic on the Schuylkill Expressway and Roosevelt Blvd. Half the people in Philadelphia were probably out doing their Christmas shopping. He was behind a big truck loaded with freshly cut Christmas trees. This truck practically stopped traffic because some of the trees had fallen off the truck. The driver had to stop to pick up the trees which had fallen off. Some of the stranded drivers were blowing their horns, and some of them were screaming obscenities.

Michael turned on the stereo of his car and played classical music to muffle the blowing of horns and the obscenities.

Finally, after twenty-five minutes, traffic started moving again.

As soon as he got to the Secula residence, he noticed the X'mas lights around the pine trees outside the porch. The windows were all lighted with Christmas candles. There was a big birthday cake on the dining room table.

"Laura, whose birthday is it today?"

"It's Dad's birthday. We went to church early this morning. On our way home, we decided to buy a birthday cake. This is one way of keeping his memory alive. Don't you think so?"

"That's nice."

Dinner was good. Everyone had their fill of Mrs. Secula's lasagna. Everyone took a second helping. Dessert was served with coffee.

Beep-Beep. Michael was beeped for an emergency. He had to leave at once. He talked to the senior resident before he left the Secula residence. There had been a train derailment in West Philadelphia, and two surgical residents were already on their way to the site of the accident. By the time Michael got there, the residents were busy sorting the passengers that had to be treated first and those that could be sent by ambulances to neighboring hospitals. There were ten people who were injured. Two people had died; their bodies were mangled because they had been thrown out the train as a result of the sudden impact of the derailment.

Television reporters and crews were busy interviewing the unhurt passengers. The passengers who had been hurt were moaning and groaning; some of them looked frightened, some of them were crying and screaming for help. The site of the accident seemed to be surrounded by a valley of human suffering. The doctors were being followed around by T.V. reporters. It was past midnight when the last derailment victim left the site of the accident. His family was going to take him home. The doctors were exhausted, but relieved and quite fulfilled that they were able to do their best in this most untenable circumstance.

"What a relief! Finally, we were able to put into good use all those disaster drills which we have been staging."

"Thank God, there were not that many casualties and deaths. My heart goes out to each and every one of the victims' loved ones. They must be in shock."

Michael went back to the hospital. There were still derailment victims waiting to be seen in the accident ward. He helped the doctors in the accident ward, and the last victim was seen at 5:00 a.m. Two male victims had to have open reduction of their fractures in the operating room. One female victim, fortyish and heavyset, had a massive heart attack while waiting to be seen in the emergency room. She was coded, revived, and resting comfortably in the Coronary Care Unit. Her harrowing experience probably triggered her heart attack.

Michael tried to get some sleep before his eight o'clock case. He had to scrub with the senior resident in the morning for an embolectomy case.

He woke up around 6:45 a.m. He dropped by Charlie's room on his way to the operating room.

Charlie was already awake.

"Dr. Olsire, please don't forget to call my mother-in-law this afternoon. I'm counting on you."

"I won't. I might even take Laura with me when I go and see Mrs. Collins."

"I am glad."

Michael's operation went smoothly. He took a short nap. After lunch, he tried to call Laura. Laura was still in surgery. So, he left a message for her to call him.

Laura did not call Michael until 3:30 p.m.

"Michael, what are you up to?"

"How about coming with me to see Mrs. Collins?"

"I can't."

"Why?"

"I have to go to Smithsvale Hospital to moonlight in the surgical and medical department."

"I didn't know that."

"I was going to tell you last night, but you got called."

"How many times a week are you going to do this?"

"Twice a week on the nights I am off."

"That means I will not be able to see you at all."

"You could, if you wanted to."

"How?"

"You can moonlight in the same hospital. You can moonlight in the emergency room once a week."

"I think I might have to think about that. I worry about my liability insurance coverage. I am under the liability insurance program of the university. I do not want to jeopardize my insurance coverage. Who covers your liability insurance?"

"Smithsvale Hospital. Michael, excuse me, I have to go. I should be at Smithsvale Hospital by five o'clock. Call me when you get back from Mrs. Collins' house."

"I will."

"Be careful driving."

"Thank you."

Michael called up Mrs. Collins. She answered the phone and said, "Patty is not home from work yet. I am by myself. Everyone should be home soon. Do you want to leave a message for Patty?"

Michael said, "No, I would like to come and visit you."

"I would be delighted. What time are you going to come?"

"I would like to come now."

"That would be fine. You can stay for dinner, too."

It took Michael an hour to get to Germantown. The Schuylkill Expressway traffic was not moving. By the time he arrived at Vestar St., there was hardly a place to park; so, he parked across the street in a hospital lot.

Mrs. Collins did not tell Patty or the girls that Michael Olsire was coming. Patty and the girls had gone to the university hospital to visit Charlie.

The food was still on the table when Michael arrived. Mrs. Collins, who had been wheelchair confined for a while, was very handy with her wheelchair. She put the food on the table. She motioned Michael to sit across from her at the dinner table. Michael tried to help

Mrs. Collins with her wheelchair, but she was way ahead of him. Michael just stood there watching her and smiled.

"You are such an amazing lady. So independent."

"I have to be. I am by myself the whole day. I have to help myself. Dr. Olsire, let's eat. I am glad you could come and see me. Did Charlie send you here?"

"Not exactly. I had planned to come here and talk to you personally about Charlie's illness, but I had to come sooner than I thought because Charlie's condition is rapidly deteriorating. Did Patty tell you what's wrong with Charlie?"

"Not exactly. She told me that Charlie has a viral condition which could be fatal."

"Have you ever heard of AIDS?"

"Yes. I have seen people talk about it on T.V. I know from watching T.V. that it is a very controversial subject. Where do you think Charlie got it from?"

"Probably from drug abuse."

"How do you know?"

"Charlie got hooked up with drugs in the street, not by choice but by necessity. A legal powerhouse was going to turn Charlie and his friends in to the police if they did not sell drugs for him."

"I see. How did you meet Charlie?"

"In the accident ward of University Hospital. We did an emergency splenectomy on him. We became friends from then on."

"You have given so much of yourself to my family. I hope we will be able to repay you in the future."

"Don't worry about it, Mrs. Collins. The reason I came here is to talk to you about Charlie and how badly he feels for whatever unhappiness he has caused you and Patty. He does not have that much time left. I wish you and Charlie would bury the hatchet and make up. You will make him feel good, and, at least, it will give him peace of mind. What do you think, Mrs. Collins?"

"I have already forgiven Charlie, but I have not yet visited him in the hospital."

"Do you want to visit him tonight? I can take you there myself. It would surprise everyone."

"But it is too much for you to do this for me."

"I don't think so. It's much easier for me than for Patty. I will just wheel you down the ramp to my car. What do you say, Mrs. Collins?"

"How can I refuse such an offer from a nice doctor like you?"

Michael wheeled Mrs. Collins down the ramp of her porch. Then, he lifted her out of the wheelchair and into the front seat of his car. He put the wheelchair into his trunk. He sped away towards the Schuylkill and reached the hospital in no time.

As soon as they reached the lobby of the hospital, Michael requested the Security Guard to watch Mrs. Collins while he parked his car in the doctors' parking lot.

Michael wheeled Mrs. Collins to the fourth floor where Charlie was. He carefully opened Charlie's door. Everyone was surprised to see Mrs. Collins. Michael pushed Mrs. Collins' wheelchair near Charlie's bed. Charlie tried to reach Mrs. Collins so he could hug her, but he was too weak. Instead, he reached for her hand and squeezed it.

Charlie exclaimed, "Thanks, Mom," and started sobbing. "Thank you for caring and coming."

"Charlie, you have to thank Dr. Olsire. He came to visit me today. He was the one who explained everything to me. He went out of his way to do what was not even expected of him. He cares a lot about you, Charlie. He is your friend."

Everyone was listening to the interaction between Charlie and Mrs. Collins.

"Mom, you have made me very happy," said Patty.

"Thank you, Grandmom. You really have lifted Dad's spirit with your visit."

Everyone hugged Mrs. Collins. Dr. Olsire, beaming with joy, just watched.

"Do any of you want something to drink?"

"Dr. Olsire, we should be buying you a drink. But thanks anyway. We will be leaving soon. Visiting hours are almost over."

"I will take Mrs. Collins home. You can follow us. It is easier for me to push her wheelchair onto the ramp of your house."

"Thank you, Dr. Olsire."

As soon as they arrived at Vestar St., Michael took the wheelchair from his trunk. He lifted Mrs. Collins out of the car and into the wheelchair. Patty and the girls got out of their car.

As soon as he had wheeled Mrs. Collins up to the porch, he said goodbye to everyone. "I have to go now. I have to drop by Smithsvale Hospital to see how Laura is doing."

CHAPTER XI

Michael arrived at Smithsvale Hospital. The accident ward was packed with patients. The Triage area was very busy, too. He went to the accident ward to have Laura paged. Laura could not come to the phone so Michael went to the telemetry unit where Laura was. Laura was in the hallway with two other doctors and two nurses. They were wheeling two dead patients to the morgue of the hospital.

When Laura saw Michael, she called him.

"Laura, what happened to these two patients?"

"These two patients not only lived in the same neighborhood, they also occupied the same hospital room. Mrs. White was coded. We were trying to resuscitate her. Mrs. Hill started complaining of chest pains so we told her to relax. A few minutes later, there was silence. When we failed to revive Mrs. White, we opened Mrs. Hill's drape. She was also dead. It's so frustrating."

Before Laura could finish talking, she was paged STAT to the third floor medical building.

By the time she got to the floor, the patient was lying in a pool of blood. This patient had threatened to commit suicide because he did not want to be hooked up to a machine all his life. He was very depressed. The nurses thought he was going to jump out the window. They brought him close to the nurses' station so he could be watched closely. There was one nurse and two nurse's aides on the floor with eighteen patients. The patient became furious and pulled his shunt; the artery pulsated and blood spurted all over the walls. It was morbid.

Laura was exhausted and frustrated. Michael felt sorry for her.

"Laura, do you really want to continue doing this kind of moonlighting job?"

"I am not sure now. I signed for six nights of night duty. I will only do this until December 23rd; then I might just work in the accident ward."

"Why do you have to do this?"

"I want to help Mom pay some bills. Real estate taxes and income tax time are coming. I also have to pay off my student loan. I will survive these stresses. I will just have to eat well and get as much rest as I can."

"I brought you something to eat."

"Michael, I have to call all the attending physicians of these three dead patients. Then we can go to the Snack Bar. What did you bring, Michael?"

"I brought you a fresh turkey sandwich and a Tastykake."

"Thank you, I'm really starved. I have not had dinner. As soon as I arrived, I had to scrub in the operating room because the O.R. nurse could not get the surgical assistant. The O.R. nurse asked if I would scrub, so I did. Michael, it's getting late. It's almost eleven o'clock. I think you better go back to the university. I will talk to you tomorrow."

"I will call you later."

"Alright, and thank you for the sandwich and Tastykake, and for thinking of me."

As soon as Michael got home, he called Laura.

He was not able to talk to her because she was scrubbed in the operating room.

The next day, Michael called Laura. Still he could not talk to her because she was scrubbed the whole day. It was almost seven in the evening when Laura got out of the operating room. She was so exhausted that she fell asleep in her call room.

Michael was worried that something might have happened to her because she was not answering her page. He called Laura's house. Mrs. Secula answered.

"Laura is still at the hospital. She will sleep first before she comes home. She is very tired from working at Smithsvale. I wish you would talk to her about stopping this moonlighting job."

"Mrs. Secula, I don't think she will listen to me. She already told me that she needs to moonlight. Please tell her I called. I will be waiting for her call."

"Good night, Michael."

"Good night, Mrs. Secula."

CHAPTER XII

Laura returned Michael's call as soon as she came home.

"Laura, I have good news for you. My hepatitis and Western Blot tests are both negative."

"I am so happy for you."

"Now, this calls for a celebration! When can we go out to dinner?"

"We can go out before Christmas, if you are not on call. There should be no problem with your schedule since you are a fellow. I will try to change with another resident on December 23rd."

"But I think it would be better if we went out on the 24th rather than the 23rd. So, just keep your schedule the way it is."

"Whatever you say, Michael."

"I will be talking to you tomorrow. Are you going to be on call at Smithsvale Hospital tomorrow?"

"Yes, please don't bring me any more food. I will just buy a sandwich before I leave the hospital."

"May I come down to see you in case you are not busy?"

"Please call me first."

"Will do."

Laura was very busy at Smithsvale Hospital the next night. It was snowing, and the roads were very icy. There were many accidents. One young lady was brought to the hospital DOA after her car crashed into a tree due to the icy road. The cops had a hard time getting her out of the wrecked car. The car was practically totalled. Laura had several admissions to the Coronary Care Unit. As soon as she finished writing the orders on her new admissions and notifying the attending physicians, she called Michael.

"Michael, please don't come. The roads are icy and driving is treacherous."

"Thank you for your concern. I hope you're not busy."

"I hope so, too. About five pregnant patients have just been admitted. Three of them are in active labor. If one or two of these patients are sectioned, I will have to scrub. I don't think the surgical assistant will be able to drive in with this kind of weather. Michael, I have to go now. I want to get some sleep before I get busy."

"Sweet dreams."

"You, too,"

As soon as Laura arrived at her call room, the phone was already ringing. The delivery room nurse called her to do a history and physical examination on a patient with non-reassuring fetal heartbeat. Laura went to the delivery room immediately. By the time she arrived in the delivery room, the patient was already being wheeled into the Caesarean section room. The fetal heartbeat dropped suddenly after the Epidural anaesthesia was injected. The fetal heartbeat never recovered to normal pattern. Laura had to scrub. At delivery, the baby was limp and the apgar was five. The baby was resuscitated by the neonatologist. The baby perked up after five minutes. The apgar became eight. There had been a tight cord around the baby's neck. The father was called to the delivery room to see the baby; the father was elated. There was an immediate bonding between the baby and the parents.

Laura went back to her call room after she finished assisting with the Caesarean section. She was opening the door when her phone rang again. It was a STAT call from the delivery room. She was needed to scrub for another Caesarean section.

The patient was a 32-year-old primigravida with previously diagnosed placenta praevia. Her HMO insurance had denied an extension of her stay in the hospital two weeks ago. She had been sent home still spotting whenever she moved. She had been rushed to the hospital by the ambulance practically in shock because of hemorrhage with severe abdominal pain. Also, the husband had not been able to get through to the ambulance immediately. He was frantically calling while at the same time helplessly watching his wife practically bleed to death. The dispatcher had a hard time understanding him, too. As soon as the ambulance had reached the hospital, the emergency room physician had called the delivery room to be ready for a shocky patient. The patient's hemoglobin was 8.5 grams. The platelet count was 110,000 per cubic mm.; the fibrinogen level was 150 mg. The patient was immediately typed and crossed. Albumin solution was maintaining her blood volume. The fetal heartbeat was no longer audible. Three units of blood had to be pumped into the patient before anaesthesia could be started. The patient did not stop bleeding even after the surgery and blood transfusion. STAT hemorrhagic studies were repeated, and they were all abnormal. The fibrinogen level was zero. The platelet count was only 38,000. The patient was bleeding from all over her body cavities. Urine showed hematuria. Three hours later, the patient had anuria (no urine output) and renal shutdown. The patient died thirty minutes after renal shutdown.

There was so much chaos in the delivery room. Everyone was busy trying to save the patient, but to no avail.

Laura felt bad for the woman who had died. She could see the somber, sunken, pale white face and pained expression of the bereaved widower. She felt so bad that she was not able to talk to him to tell him how sorry she was that this had to happen to his wife. The situation seemed unbearable to everyone. Two lives lost because the insurance company had wanted to make more profit, and because the doctor had not stood up for his patient.

Laura woke up early, but could hardly get out of the bed in her call room. She was exhausted and frustrated. She quickly took a shower, got dressed, and ran to the hospital cafeteria for a quick cup of coffee.

It was almost seven in the morning, and the traffic on the Schuylkill Expressway was not moving. Laura was getting fidgety. Her first case in the operating room was at 8:00 a.m. Finally, the traffic started moving, and she arrived at Northend Hospital in due time. She made a quick round just to see if there were patients who needed urgent attention or orders to be changed or rewritten. Done by eight, she rushed to the operating room.

Her first patient was a 56-year-old lady readmitted for revision of her colostomy and bowel resection. She had been following this woman's progress for several months. The operation went smoothly.

As soon as Laura finished her operation, she went up to the surgical floor to await the arrival of her next patient for localization biopsy of a 5 mm. density on her right breast.

Laura was paged in the operating room for her breast biopsy case. This pleasant 45-year-old lady was quite upset. She went to the doctor every six months, and the mammogram had shown the 5 mm. density just one week ago. Laura was able to biopsy the density, and a frozen section revealed a benign lesion to the delight of the patient and Laura.

It was already 3:30 p.m. by the time she finished in the surgical clinic.

She went back to the surgical ward to work-up and pre-op her admission scheduled for surgery in the morning.

By 5:30 p.m., she was done. She rushed home because she had to take her mother to the mall. Christmas decorations and music were all over the place. The mall was crowded since there were only two weeks left before Christmas. All the stores at the Northeast Mall were packed. All of a sudden, people were running away from the center of the mall. Laura heard a muffled gunshot.

"Mom, let's stay inside the store until everything calms down. There might be more shooting."

Inside the store, they could hear the police siren.

After forty-five minutes, everything was back to normal. Laura and Mrs. Secula resumed their shopping.

It was almost 10:30 p.m. when they arrived home. The phone was ringing. Jeanie was not home yet. By the time Laura picked up the phone, the caller had hung up.

"It might have been Michael."

He will call back if he really wants to talk to me."

RING===RING===RING.

"Laura, how are you? I have been trying to call you for hours. How was your duty at Smithsvale Hospital?"

"It was catastrophic. They had a maternal death there. An HMO insurance patient. It was terrible. I will never forget the pain and anguish of the family. It is so unconscionable that doctors would let the government and the insurance companies dictate their medical practice at the expense of patients' lives. Why don't they educate their patients about HMO's fraudulent advertising and the financial incentives involved? Aren't these doctors guilty of fraud and conspiracy when they don't tell their patients that they get bonuses if they do less testing, less referral to specialists, and if they delay or deny their hospitalization admissions?"

"Everything you say is true. Organized medicine is in trouble. We have not really policed our profession. There is still conspiracy of silence. We are rugged individualists and very disorganized. That is why we can't get anywhere with politicians. The politicians are trying to decrease the federal deficit, so they have selectively discriminated against us and the hospitals. They treat us like criminals when we try to provide the best care for our elderly patients. If the diagnosis does not fall under the CPT Code, the government refuses to pay the bill. Healthcare rationing is already well-entrenched in the form of HMO insurance. But HMO is not really quality patient care because it is profit motivated. They would not last, though, if they started insuring the elderly and the poor because they would start losing more money."

"I think so, too."

"Will I be able to see you tomorrow?"

"I am going to work at Smithsvale."

"I will call you then."

"Alright, good night."

Laura was in the hospital by 7:00 a.m. the next day. She wanted to make rounds on all the post-operative patients. She was worried that she might not have enough time to see them all in the afternoon after her clinic. She had to start working at Smithsvale Hospital at 6:00 p.m.

By the time she arrived at Smithsvale Hospital, she already had two patients for histories and physicals who were left-overs from that day's admission. One lady waiting for a bed in the telemetry unit had unstable angina. Another patient was a transfer from a nursing home. This lady had had a stroke and had developed bilateral lobe pneumonia. She was quite confused and could not remember where the nursing home was located. Laura had a difficult time talking to her. She did not have any family member with her. Laura could not believe the huge decubitus ulcers on her lower back. She had been in the nursing home for only three weeks! Her muscle tone was also poor. This lady was probably not eating enough protein. Laura started the patient's intravenous fluids with intravenous medications.

Code 1=== Code 1=== Code 1=== Room 231

Laura excused herself and told the elderly patient that she would be back later.

Laura ran towards the telemetry unit. The code had been taken care of by the other residents on duty. The patient was resuscitated and the attending physician was immediately notified at home.

The cardiologist came to the coronary care unit without any delay. By the time he arrived, the patient had become more responsive. He just had to be monitored carefully. His family was notified, too. The cardiologist took the family aside and explained to them what was going on.

After everything was under control, Laura went back to see the elderly lady she had admitted an hour ago. The lady was already sleeping peacefully so she did not bother her anymore.

As soon as she went back to her room to get some sleep, her phone rang. It was Michael.

"Laura, I have more news for you. Charlie is not doing well. His T-cells are down to 180 per cubic mm. of blood. Another man who used to share a needle with Charlie was admitted with tunnelling ulcers in his buttocks. Tom Wittle placed him on AZT. He has no lung findings, though. I am quite worried. I could be positive anytime."

"Michael, get some sleep. You will be fine. Think positive."

"I hope so. Will I be able to see you tomorrow?"

"I will be on call at the university. You can drop by if I'm not busy."

"I will do that. I am going to visit Charlie before I take off. I have to talk to Charlie's family about his condition. I have to call Mrs. Collins tomorrow. I want to explain to her what's going on. She is counting on me."

"Michael, you really get involved with your patients."

"They are just my friends. I have known Charlie for almost a year now. I feel, though, that we have known each other for years. He always looks forward to seeing me."

"I think so, too. You have spoiled him and his family. I hope they appreciate what you are trying to do for them."

"I just do it because I like to do it. That's what medicine is all about. I know you feel as I do when it comes to patient care. Otherwise, you would not get so upset when you see patients being ripped off by the doctors whom they trust."

"You win this time. Tell Charlie I said, 'hello.' I will try to see him next time I am off."

"That would be nice."

"Michael, I want to get some sleep before I get called again. I have already had two admissions and a code. Hopefully, I won't get called in an obstetrical emergency."

"I will let you go now. Talk to you tomorrow. Good night."

At 3:00 a.m., Laura was called again in another code. By the time she got to the floor, the patient had already expired. This was an elderly lady in the oncology unit with brain metastasis. She had developed generalized convulsive seizures and then had stopped breathing.

"My God, someone dies everytime I come to work at this hospital. I must be a jinx."

Laura went back to her call room to try to get some sleep. She had to wake up early and leave by 6:00 a.m. to catch up with the surgical grand round at Northend.

When Laura left Smithsvale, she couldn't find her car in the parking lot. She paged the security guard. The security guard couldn't come immediately because he was trying to overcome a patient in the mental health unit who had tried to beat up other patients. He had punched the head nurse and nurse supervisor. Both were now being treated in the accident ward.

Laura tried to call Jeanie at home, but she had already left for work. So she called Michael.

"Laura, you sound so upset."

"I am. Somebody stole my car in the doctor's parking lot. I have already called the police to report the theft. Do you think you would have enough time to pick me up and take me to work?"

"I will be there as soon as possible. I will tell the chief resident to take over the conference."

"Thank you. I knew I could count on you."

Michael was at Smithsvale Hospital in thirty minutes. He felt so sorry for Laura. She looked haggard and was about to burst into tears any minute. He put his arms around her shoulders and said, "Don't worry. They will find your car, and, if not, the insurance company will pay the book value."

"Michael, my car is already old and has practically no book value."

"Then just buy a second-hand car."

"I will have to."

They reached Northend Hospital in no time. Laura thanked Michael and ran towards the surgical building.

Everyone looked at Laura when she arrived at the meeting. The grand round was about to be finished. After the grand round was over, Laura asked to be excused. She had to call the police to see if they had any leads on her car.

The officer at Precinct 12 said, "No. I don't think we will ever find out who stole your car. Car thieves usually chop up the cars they steal and sell the parts of the car for more money."

"I have to get another car then."

"I think that's a good idea. I will call you if anything comes up."

"Thank you very much. Have a nice day."

"You, too."

Laura went down to the operating room to operate on a young boy with acute appendicitis. This young boy had been seen in another hospital but had not been admitted because he had no insurance. The emergency room physician from the other hospital had not even bothered to call the emergency room doctor at Northend Hospital about the patient. He just told the mother to take a taxi and go to the emergency room of Northend Hospital.

Laura was furious when she found this out from the mother. She called the resident and told him off.

"Do you know that you could be guilty of a federal offense with a fine of $50,000.00? You would jeopardize the medicare participation of your hospital, too!"

The emergency room resident said, "I'm sorry. I will not do this again."

"I hope so because, the next time you do this to a patient, I will be the one who reports you to the proper authorities."

"Thank you."

Laura talked to the mother of the patient to appease her. "Your son will be fine. He should be out of bed by tomorrow morning. Is there anything I can do for you? If you want to get something to eat, you can go to the cafeteria or the social spot."

"Thank you, Dr. Secula."

"If there is anything I can do for you, don't hesitate to call me."

"Thanks again, doctor."

Laura called Precinct 12 again. Still no news about her car.

"I guess I have to accept it. I might as well look for another car."

Laura called up Michael.

"Michael, do you think you could take me to a second-hand car dealer tomorrow? Now, don't feel obligated."

"Yes, I can, but it won't be until after Journal Club. I will meet you at 7:00 p.m. in the parking lot of your hospital."

"Thanks."

Michael was on time. He was at the door of the hospital lobby by 7:00 p.m., but Laura was not there. He got out of his car and requested the information desk to page Laura. Laura was still in the operating room. She was assisting the senior resident in an emergency case. It was a ruptured abdominal aneurysm according to the nurse who answered the phone for Laura.

Michael requested the nurse to ask Laura if she wanted him to wait until she was done.

Laura said, "Yes. Please tell him I will be down as soon as we get done. Tell him that we are already closing the peritoneum. Thank you."

Laura came down to the lobby as soon as she was finished in the operating room.

"You look tired."

"I'm not only tired, I am starved, too."

"I brought you some dinner. I knew you must have forgotten to eat today. You were so engrossed with your lost car."

"You are a mind reader! Thank you for thinking of me."

"Do you still want to go to the second-hand dealer lot?"

"No, it's already eight-thirty. The lot closes at nine. So, by the time we get there, the lot will be ready to close. I am just going to sleep in my call room. We have early rounds tomorrow. Do you want to share this sandwich with me?"

"No, I am full. I will get you a soda at the social spot. I will see you tomorrow. We can go to the second-hand car lot and look for a car."

"I can't go tomorrow. I have to leave early before three. I have to apply for a car loan. I want to get the car as soon as possible. I have four more work nights at Smithsvale Hospital. I would rather work in the emergency room, though. I think I will apply at Southern Hospital."

Beep, Beep - Michael was beeped by the hospital. It was an emergency.

"Laura, I have to leave. I will call you later."

CHAPTER XIII

As soon as Michael got to the hospital door, he heard a Code 1 for Room 443. Michael rushed to the elevator, but it was stuck on the ground floor. He ran through the exit door up to the fourth floor. He saw that everyone was going towards Charlie's room. By the time he entered the room, Charlie was already in cardiac arrest and could not be resuscitated. Michael was misty-eyed. He had gotten so involved with Charlie that he felt he had lost one of his relatives.

"Tom, did Mrs. Singleton come here tonight?"

"I don't know, Michael. I saw Charlie at four, and no visitors were here at that time."

"I saw Charlie at six, and he was talking to me about getting Christmas presents for his family. I have to call Patty Singleton and tell her the bad news."

Michael went to the nurses' desk and called Patty.

"Patty, how are you?"

"I am fine, Dr. Olsire. It's kind of late for you to call me. Did something happen to Charlie?"

"I am sorry to tell you, but Charlie went into cardiac arrest, and we could not revive him. It was unexpected. Charlie has never complained of chest pain in the past except for that pulmonary embolism. This is what we call sudden cardiac death."

Patty started sobbing. "We had been doing so well with our relationship, and this has to happen. I'm going to wake up Kathy and Michelle. We will be there as soon as we can."

"I will be waiting for you in Charlie's room. Don't get upset if you see many people inside the room. Each one of them has a job to do."

"I won't."

As soon as the elevator stopped on the fourth floor, Michael walked briskly towards its door. Patty and her girls were in it. They all looked so sad, as if the weight of the world had fallen on their shoulders. Michael hugged each of them and tried to console them. He took them to Charlie's room. Patty and the girls said their final goodbye to Charlie. Each of them kissed Charlie before his body was covered with white linen and transferred to a stretcher. His body was brought down to the morgue.

Michael talked to Patty about the funeral home arrangements. He explained to Patty about the special precautions to be used. Patty understood. She was going to have Charlie's body cremated.

"I have to tell Mom when we arrive home. I am just glad that Mom and Charlie reconciled before he died."

"I am, too. Let's go to the coffee shop before you go home. I will get you some coffee. I don't want you falling asleep while driving. Let me know about any memorial services that you will have for Charlie."

"I will only have a requiem mass for Charlie."

"I will try to be there, and probably Laura will come with me, too."

Michael accompanied Patty and her girls to the exit door of the hospital and walked them to the parking lot.

"Thank you so much, Dr. Olsire."

"Anytime, and, if there is anything I can do for you, don't hesitate to call me."

"I won't. Good night."

Michael went to his room and called Laura, "I have bad news for you. Charlie died about two hours ago. He went into cardiac arrest. We could not revive him."

"I am sorry to hear that. How is his family taking it?"

"Very well. They should be fine. I will let you know about the requiem mass."

"Alright. I would like to go if I am not tied up."

"I will talk to you tomorrow night. Good night."

The next night, Michael called Laura at seven. No answer. He called her call room. No answer. He called her at Smithsvale Hospital. No answer.

It was now eight, and Michael had not succeeded in locating Laura, Mrs. Secula, or Jeanie.

At nine, he called Laura at Northend Hospital. He was told that Laura had been rushed to the ICU unconscious. She had been mugged by three male teenagers while waiting for a ride from her sister.

Michael was so upset that he said to himself, "If something happens to Laura, I will never be able to forgive myself. I should have offered to take her to the bank instead of having her sister do it."

Michael practically flew to Northend Hospital. He didn't care whether he got a speeding ticket. What mattered to him at this time was to be with Laura.

Laura was already down at the Radiology Department for a CAT Scan when Michael arrived.

Mrs. Secula and Jeanie were sitting and crying in the waiting room. Michael hugged both of them. He started crying, too.

The radiology resident came in to read the brain scan. Michael wiped his tears and went over to the radiologist office. He introduced himself. They went over the films. The CAT Scan was negative; there was no evidence of hemorrhage.

Michael went inside the CAT Scan room to see how Laura was doing. Laura was trying to open her eyes. Michael squeezed her left hand, and he could see the grimace and arching of her arms. Michael felt relieved.

"Laura, I thought I was going to lose you."

Laura moaned, "No chance."

"I am going to the waiting room now to tell your Mom and Jeanie that everything is fine."

Michael left the Cat Scan room and explained to Mrs. Secula and Jeanie that Laura was doing well.

"Her brain was shaken by the mugging, but she will be fine."

Laura was brought back to the ICU.

Michael, Mrs. Secula, and Jeanie were allowed to visit her in her room for only fifteen minutes. They were told by the nurse that Laura needed to rest and sleep.

The three of them left together. Michael walked them to their car just to be sure they were safe.

"Michael, do you want to come home with us and get something to eat?"

"Thank you, but I feel exhausted by all this commotion. I am just glad Laura is fine. Good night."

As soon as Michael arrived at his apartment, he called Patty.

"How are you, the kids, and Mrs. Collins?"

"We are fine and coping very well."

"When will the requiem mass be held?"

"This coming Saturday."

"I will try to be there. Laura should be home by then."

"What's happened to Dr. Secula?"

"She was mugged in front of Northend Hospital while waiting for her sister to pick her up."
"I hope she is okay."
"She will do well. Is there anything I can do for you?"
"Nothing that I can think of."
"May I talk to Mrs. Collins?"
"Sure. I will put her on the phone."
"Mrs. Collins, how are you?"
"I am doing well, thank you. I am just glad Charlie and I made up before he died."
"I am glad, too. I will be seeing you soon. Take care."
"Bye, Dr. Olsire."
As soon as Michael hung up, he fell asleep. He was exhausted by the stress of Laura's accident.
The next morning Michael called the ICU of Northend Hospital to ask about Laura's condition. According to the nurse in charge of Laura, she had had a restful sleep. The nurse intended to try to get Laura out of bed today. If she could get out of bed, she would be transferred to the regular floor that afternoon.
Michael requested the nurse to tell Laura that he had called.
"I will tell her. It should make her feel good that someone cares so much about her as you do."
"Thank you."
Laura was still on intravenous fluids. Miss Walters helped her get out of bed. She barely made six steps when she started feeling dizzy. Miss Walters had to put Laura back in bed.
"Dr. Secula, please rest for a couple of hours. I will try to get you out of bed later on, after lunch."
"Thank you for your patience. Could you please call Dr. Olsire at this number? Tell him I must talk to him."
Miss Walters called Dr. Olsire, but he was scrubbed in the operating room.
"I left the message with the operating room nurse. He is going to call here as soon as he is done with his case. I will put you in a wheelchair later so that, in case he calls, you will be able to talk to him on the phone."
"You are so nice and thoughtful."
"In the meantime, get some rest. I am going to bathe the patient in the next room."
"Thank you, Miss Walters."
Two hours later, Michael was on the phone. "What is going on, Miss Walters?"
"Hold on please. I will get Dr. Secula."
"Michael, how are you?"
"I am fine now that I know you are doing better and have made a lot of progress since last night."
"Could you please do me a favor?"
"Of course."
"Could you call the Medical Director at Smithsvale Hospital and tell him that I will not be able to work Thursday and Friday?"
"I will gladly do that. I don't think you will be discharged sooner than Saturday."
"I don't think so either."
"Do you want to attend the requiem mass for Charlie if you are discharged Saturday?"
"That would be nice."
"So, tell your Mom and Jeanie that I will pick you up from the hospital on Saturday."
"That will be fine. Mom and Jeanie can sleep in late that day."

"The church is not out of the way. It will be at Miraculous Medal Church on Chelten Ave. Do you want me to bring you something to eat tonight?"

"No, thank you. I am still on intravenous fluids. I still get nauseated and dizzy when I get up and walk."

"I will see you tonight. I will give the Medical Director at Smithsvale a call as soon as I hang up."

"Thanks, Michael. I knew I could depend on you."

"You bet."

The Medical Director at Smithsvale Hospital tried to give Michael a hard time.

"This is such short notice."

"I know, but unexpected accidents happen. Dr. Secula is still in the ICU of Northend Hospital. She is still unable to walk without getting nauseous and dizzy. Today is only Tuesday. I think this is enough notice to get a replacement for her."

"I will try to call other moonlighters. If I can't get anyone to replace her, would you be able to help me out?"

"I will ask my residents if anyone is interested. Please give me a call as soon as you find out. I am sure Dr. Secula feels bad that she has to impose on other people. Please leave the message with my answering machine. I will call you back as soon as I get home tonight. Thank you."

"Thank you for calling."

Michael went back to the operating room. He did not finish operating until after five-thirty in the evening. He went to the cafeteria to get some dinner.

By seven, he was already on his way to Northend Hospital. As soon as he arrived in the ICU, he saw Laura trying to get up on her own. Suddenly, she fell to the floor face down with the intravenous fluid pole hitting the back of her head. She became unconscious.

"Laura! Laura! Nurse! Nurse! Please call a code."

Everyone rushed to Laura's room. Michael got out of the way. He looked pale and terrified.

"My God, what is going on with Laura?"

In ten minutes, Laura was revived. Everyone left her room.

Michael asked the nurse's permission to see Laura's medication card and the medicine drawer. Laura had been given Diazepam (Valium), thirty minutes before she fell.

Michael requested the nurse to call Laura's doctor. He was furious that Laura was given generic drugs without her knowledge and consent.

The nurse called the doctor. There was no answer.

"Please call him at home."

"He does not want to be called at home directly. He wants us to call the answering service first."

"You are not allowed to call him at his home?"

"No."

"Suppose it is an emergency? It would be a waste of time to wait for the answering service. Don't you think so?"

As the nurse dialed the doctor's service, she said, "The nursing staff does. But, doctors get away with the same restriction that they impose on nurses most of the time. I can't get through to the answering service."

"I have to see how Laura is doing."

"I will try the answering service again."

"Please do."

Michael returned to Laura's room.

"Laura, how are you feeling?"

"I am feeling better. I would rather not take any drugs if they are generic. I lost my balance. I thought I was walking in space."

"Just tell the nurses. Then they can relay the message to Dr. Jay."

"I will."

The nurse came in and said, "I could not get Dr. Jay. His answering service put me on hold for ten minutes. I hung up."

"Don't call him anymore. I will be fine. He will probably transfer me to the regular floor tomorrow. May I have a couple of Tylenol, please?"

"I will get them for you. Is there anything you need before I start giving out medications?"

"I think I will feel fine with just the Tylenol. Thank you. You are in a pensive mood, Michael. What's wrong?"

"Nothing. I am just thinking of Patty Singleton, her kids, and her disabled mother. She must be so overwhelmed right now."

"I think so, too. That poor soul."

"Do you think you will be able to eat regular food tomorrow?"

"I don't know yet. I don't know whether he will stop the intravenous fluids. I still get a little nauseous when I get up. We will see."

"Just give me a call if you want me to bring something for you."

"I will do that. Mom and Jeanie had just left before I fell. They had to do their last minute Christmas shopping."

"I have to go now." Michael leaned towards Laura and took her hands. "Take care. Be sure you check the medications before you take them."

"I will."

As soon as Michael arrived at his apartment, he saw the answering machine blinking. He turned it on to listen to the messages.

"Dr. Olsire, I am sorry to tell you that I could not get any replacement for Laura. Please help me out. Maybe one of your residents would like to make extra money working for two nights."

Michael called the Medical Director of Smithsvale.

"Dr. Sanders, I got your message. I will try to ask my residents at the university. But, if I can't get any replacement, I will work the two nights that Dr. Secula is supposed to work."

"Thank you, Dr. Olsire. Will I hear from you tomorrow?"

"I will be able to give you a definite answer by twelve noon."

"Good night."

As soon as Michael hung up, he called Patty Singleton.

"How are you? How is everyone?"

"So far we are doing fine. How is Dr. Secula?"

"She is doing better. She should be ready to be discharged Saturday. I will pick her up early Saturday. We will attend the requiem mass for Charlie."

"Thank you, Dr. Olsire."

Michael called several residents, but none of them could work for Laura. Michael could not sleep well. So, he got up and took out his florigraphy notebook.

"This notebook is almost filled up. I must make my move soon. Probably, I should finish filling it up tonight so that I can have it gift-wrapped for her for Christmas."

Michael woke up early. He had breakfast at the cafeteria. After breakfast, he called up the ICU at Northend Hospital to see what time Laura was going to be transferred to the regular room.

"Laura is still sleeping. The neurosurgeon has not made rounds yet. Could you call back at eleven o'clock?" asked the nurse.

"I will be in the operating room, but I will call as soon as I am finished. I want to talk to Laura before I go to Smithsvale Hospital tonight."

"I will give her the message."

Michael scrubbed with the chief resident. The cholecystectomy and exploration of the common duct went well. The patient had a lot of small stones which had not been visualized by Ultrasound or X-Ray.

"I am glad we decided to operate on her, Dr. Olsire."

"I am, too. Otherwise, we could have jeopardized her liver if we had waited too long. We are going to have our grand round now. What cases are you presenting?"

"I am going to present a case of Necrotizing Fasciitis (bacterial growth in subcutaneous tissues), post-appendectomy," said Dr. Auerglass.

"How long after surgery did the patient manifest symptoms?"

"Three days after surgery. He was discharged forty-eight hours after an appendectomy. The next day he did not feel well. The wife stated that the incision looked red and that there were crepitations when she tried to squeeze the incision to see if there was pus. The wife called the doctor, but she could not get through to his office. She kept on calling. Finally, the answering service took the message. The surgeon was already off, and someone else was covering for him. She called the covering surgeon and explained to him her fears of sepsis.

"He told her to put warm soaks on the reddened area and to call back the next day.

"The next day never came. She had to rush her husband to our accident ward after talking to the covering surgeon. Her husband was already moribund when they arrived at the accident ward. His skin was ashen gray. He was jaundiced. He was practically in septic shock. His pulse rate was 110. We immediately put in an intravenous line and a Swan-Ganz line. Garamycin and Solu-Medrol were immediately given intravenously. His output was monitored with a catheter. We rushed him to the operating room for debridement of necrotic tissues as far as we could cut. The infection had extended to his perineal area. He had to be castrated. On our way to the operating room, a STAT flat plate was done. The pockets of gas had extended to the area of the scrotum. After debridement, the incision was irrigated with hydrogen peroxide. The microorganism recovered was Bacteroides Fragilis.

"The patient is doing well in the ICU, but the patient's wife is furious. She went home after her husband's surgery, turned on the television, and saw a lawyer's advertisement about medical malpractice. She made an appointment with this lawyer. She told me she was going to sue the surgeon, the covering surgeon, the hospital, and everyone involved with her husband's care for medical malpractice."

"What credentials does she have to know all these medical facts?"

"She is an Intensive Care nurse supervisor."

"What else do you know about this life-threatening infection?"

"Eighty thousand cases of death from sepsis are reported every year, but no hospital statistics on infection rate are available to the public. No one knows the number of people dying from Necrotizing Fasciitis every year. Early diagnosis is crucial for the patient and the doctor. Late diagnosis is the cause of a high mortality rate of thirty to fifty percent. This is not a new disease. It was first reported in 1871 by Jones who called it 'Hospital Gangrene.' In 1909, Fedden reported it as 'Acute Infective Gangrene.' In 1918, Pfanner reported it as 'Necrotizing Erysipelas.' Meleney, in 1924, reported it as 'Hemolytic Streptococcus Gangrene.' McCafferty and Lyons reported it in 1948 as 'Suppurative Fasciitis.'

"Some physicians are not even aware of the existence of this condition. There is another type of Necrotizing Fasciitis which is characterized by a generalized thickening of the skin of the body that could be due to an allergic reaction to a bee sting, spider bite, or yellow fragrance No. 5. There is an outstanding increase of Eosinophiles in the white count. The patient can manifest Acute Nephrotic Syndrome with malignant elevation of blood pressure. The principle of treatment is the same although the patient will get better without surgery. Biopsy of the skin should be indicated in some cases.

"In diabetics, the mortality rate is more than fifty percent. Necrotizing Fasciitis of the fetal scalp has also been reported due to fetal monitoring."

That afternoon, the surgical grand round went well without too much discussion. The resident who had managed the Necrotizing Fasciitis case successfully was congratulated.

He said, "Early recognition and diagnosis were on my side. Knowing what medical condition you are treating and why you are treating it a certain way solves fifty percent of the problem."

"I agree with you. I hope you don't see any more cases like this one. We have to be thankful the patient is young and healthy. Otherwise, it would have been catastrophic. Need I say more? I will see you all tomorrow. Are you ready for Journal Club tomorrow afternoon? Who is presenting the case?"

"Joe Dixon."

"How about starting the meeting at one in the afternoon? The cases we have tomorrow are breast biopsies only."

"That will be fine."

CHAPTER XIV

Michael called Northend Hospital to see if Laura had been transferred. Laura had been transferred to Room 201. He requested the operator to connect him with her room.

"Laura, I will not be able to see you today. I have to rush to Smithsvale Hospital. I have to be on time. I have to do several histories and physical examinations in the ICU. How was your day?"

"I was able to walk today, but I still got dizzy and nauseous. Dr. Jay wants to repeat the CAT Scan because of my fall, but I told him I would rather wait to see if I develop more cerebral symptoms. I don't want to be exposed to unnecessary radiation."

"I can't blame you. I have to go now. Rest and sleep well. I will call you tomorrow."

By the time Michael arrived at Smithsvale Hospital, a Code 1 for Room 232 was being announced on the loudspeaker. He ran towards Room 232. The room was crowded. The patient was being resuscitated by other residents and the Anaesthesia Department. An endotracheal tube was inserted to assist her respiration. This patient was a known asthmatic who had arrived at the hospital in respiratory distress. The family brought in a bag of pills they had found floating in the toilet bowl last night after the patient had moved her bowels. Her aminophylline level was 6 mcgm. while the therapeutic level was 10-20 mcgm. The tablets were not absorbed and were generic. The tablets were submitted for analysis. The members of the patient's family were very upset. They were blaming the family doctor for not putting "Brand Necessary" on the prescription blank.

Michael went out to see the family after the patient had been stabilized. He explained to them the cause of the respiratory problem.

"I will have to call your family doctor so that you can talk to him about the medical condition of your daughter."

"No need to. We are going to call the HMO office and demand a pulmonary specialist for my daughter. This has gone too far. This would not have happened if our doctor had listened to my daughter when she told him that she did not feel well with the pills he was prescribing for her. They must be generic drugs. We are not dumb. My brother works for a major brand name drug firm. I know my daughter did not get the therapeutic level of the drug because the pills were just passing through her intestines."

"I'm sorry to hear that. Please get in touch with your HMO now. I will check the list of HMO pulmonary specialists here so you can tell HMO whom you want to take care of your daughter."

"Thank you, Dr. Olsire."

Michael went down to the Admissions Office to see if there were HMO pulmonary specialists affiliated with Smithsvale Hospital. There were none. He went back to the second floor and told the patient's parents.

"We don't really know any specialists. Could you recommend a pulmonary specialist for us, please?"

Michael responded, "I don't really know any specialist here. I'll have to call my friend and ask her."

Michael called Laura at Northend Hospital.

"Laura, who among the pulmonary specialists here would you recommend?"

"Dr. Sweedle, I think, is the best one."

"I have to go now. I have to call the primary care physician so he can order the consultation for this poor patient."

Michael went back to the second floor. He talked to the parents of Deanna, the patient.

"I must get the phone number of your HMO primary care physician to get the consultation for Deanna approved by him. HMO might not pay the hospital bill if Deanna's admission is not approved by him."

"His name is Dr. Dough."

"That name sounds familiar to me. I will call him now."

Michael called Dr. Dough and introduced himself.

"Deanna Quigley was admitted in status asthmaticus. She needs a pulmonary specialist to see her. Right now, she is stabilized and hooked up to a respirator."

Dr. Dough answered, "Her family did not notify me that she was enroute to the hospital!"

"There was no time to notify you. She was in bad shape. She was coded in the hospital ICU. If you are smart, you will give the okay now and stop the run around. The patient's parents are furious with you. You are also starting to annoy me. I hope you have big liability insurance because you are risking and increasing your own liability for fraud and racketeering everytime you refuse patients' requests for specialist consultation when their lives are at risk."

"Stop telling me what to do!"

"I'm not telling you what to do! I'm trying to protect the interest of this patient who needs further respiratory function evaluation. Just remember you are betraying this patient's trust, you are increasing HMO profit, and you are also practicing against the Hippocratic Oath."

"Stop lecturing me. Get the specialist you want and I will send the approval."

"I will get Dr. Sweedle to see her. Thank you."

Michael called Dr. Sweedle's answering service and left the message that the call was an emergency. Dr. Sweedle called back in ten minutes.

"Dr. Sweedle, thank you for calling back immediately. I have a patient in the ICU, Deanna Quigley, a 22-year-old with a history of asthma since age ten. She came to the accident ward in status asthmaticus. She was coded but is now stabilized. She is on Aminophylline I.V. She was given bolus dose of intravenous steroids and is on the respirator. We are running blood PH and blood gases, and the results should be in by the time you get here. I'm going to stay in the ICU until you arrive. I have to calm down the family. They are furious with the HMO doctor for failure to refer her to a pulmonary specialist. I can't blame them."

"I could not agree more with the family. We have been seeing more deaths due to poorly treated asthmatics. The public should be educated about this problem. The patients should be educated about HMO's profit motive and financial incentives given to physicians."

"It's a shame that organized medicine has not been aggressive enough about educating the public about the HMO's."

"I know, but the government protects the HMO's because of their vested interest."

Dr. Sweedle arrived at the ICU of Smithsvale Hospital in no time. He went directly to Room 232 where Michael was waiting. He introduced himself to the parents and to Michael. He then requested the parents to wait outside the room while he was examining Deanna.

"Each of you did a magnificent job stabilizing Deanna," said Dr. Sweedle to Michael. "Did you get the rest of the laboratory studies?"

"Yes. We have two sets. Before and after resuscitation. The PH and PO2 and PCO2 are very much improved."

"She is not out of the woods yet. It must have been scary. I have seen only a few patients that presented in the emergency room this sick."

"The parents called the HMO doctor yesterday. He never called back. I'm glad they had the common sense to rush her to the emergency room."

"Will you be working here tomorrow during the day, Dr. Olsire?"

"No. I'm just relieving Dr. Secula."

"I have to talk to one of the house physicians so someone will be aware of this patient's problem."

"I think you should call Dr. Dough and tell him off. He likes to treat patients beyond the scope of his medical knowledge. He should be taught a lesson. This patient should have been referred to a pulmonary specialist from the start. He should have volunteered to refer her to a specialist if he had cared enough about his patient rather than about filling up his pocketbook with green bucks."

"I agree with you, Dr. Olsire. This type of physician is the kind whom the public would remember most. He is giving the medical profession a bad name."

"I know, and good and caring physicians are put in the same basket as the greedy and uncaring ones."

"I'm glad to have met a young physician who practices the Aesculapian-Hippocratic type of medicine. I'm going to write some orders. If you would, please check Deanna and let me know how she is doing before you go to bed and before you take off tomorrow."

"I will be glad to do that."

Michael had to call all the surgical floors to see if there was any patient who needed to have a history and physical examination done. There were only two. Before he left the ICU, he talked to Deanna's parents and reassured them. He told them that, although he would be working in the hospital for two nights only, he would still visit Deanna tomorrow. He asked them if they would like to get something to eat.

Mr. and Mrs. Quigley thanked Michael.

"I wish all doctors were like this young man. He is so caring. He just met us this afternoon. He made us feel that we have known him for years. There is nothing phony about him, either."

"I know. He told me he is a fellow at University Hospital. I'm going to ask for his address and phone number since we might need him later."

"That's a good idea."

Michael went to the fourth floor to do his histories and physical examinations.

The first patient was a diabetic man with stasis ulcer and popliteal artery insufficiency. His diabetes was out of control. He was admitted prior to surgery in order to control his diabetes.

The second patient that Michael saw was an elderly, obese lady with incarcerated umbilical hernia. She would have to be operated on tonight. She was originally scheduled for surgery the next day, but she had been admitted through the accident ward. The operating room had just called for her. The surgeon would be in shortly and Michael would have to scrub.

It was almost 11:00 p.m. when the umbilical hernia repair was finished. Michael went to the ICU to check on Deanna Quigley. Deanna's vital signs were stable. Her blood PH and blood gases were much improved. Her lungs sounded better, and her output was good.

He called Dr. Sweedle and gave him the update on Deanna's condition.

"This young lady, Deanna, is doing well. Her blood PH and blood gases are much better. Her signs are stable. I will call you again in the morning before I take off."

On his way to his call room, he met Mr. and Mrs. Quigley again. He gave them a progress report on Deanna.

"Your daughter is really doing good. I am very optimistic about her condition. She should be weaned off the respirator in a few days."

"Thank you, doctor,"

"We hope we will see you again tomorrow."

Michael was hoping that he would be able to call Laura that night, but it was too late. So, he went to sleep.

At three in the morning, his phone rang. It was a STAT page. The delivery room wanted him immediately to scrub on a Caesarean section. The patient was unregistered, and she had come in with a prolapsed cord. There was no time to wait for the anesthesiologist. The lady was operated on under local anaesthesia. After the baby was delivered and resuscitated, the anesthesiologist put the patient to sleep by crash induction. Everything went well. The husband, who was waiting nervously outside the Caesarean section room, was informed that mother and baby were both doing fine. He went to the social spot to make phone calls after he heard the good news.

By the time the Caesarean section was finished, it was almost five in the morning. Michael went to the ICU to check on Deanna Quigley. He saw her parents dozing in the waiting room. Michael checked Deanna's lungs and vital signs. Her lungs sounded better than they did last night. He ordered the blood PH and blood gases. He instructed the nurse in charge of Deanna's care to notify Dr. Sweedle of the test results as soon as they were available.

By seven in the morning, Michael was already back at the university. He was tired and sleepy. He drank two cups of coffee to keep himself going.

He tried to call Laura before going to the operating room, but the operator said that it was too early to wake up patients. It was only 7:15 a.m.

As soon as Michael got out of the operating room, he called Laura. He asked her how she was doing. "I am doing fine. I was able to walk last night without getting dizzy and nauseous. I will try to do better today. I want to go home Saturday. I have to wrap some Christmas presents, too."

"I will not be able to visit you today. I will be tied up until I am ready to go to Smithsvale Hospital. I had a very busy night. I had a patient with status asthmaticus. Her doctor is Dr. Dough. She had a hard time getting referral to a pulmonary specialist. She landed in the emergency room. Her Aminophylline level was only 6 mcgm. I think I got Dr. Dough scared. I told him that he might get sued for fraud and racketeering because of the financial incentives involved. He is the same HMO doctor who gave Patty Singleton a hard time about referring Kathy Singleton to a cardiologist."

"It serves him right. The patients need to be educated about this financial incentive. What time are you going to pick me up tomorrow?"

"I should be there by nine in the morning."

"I am sure Dr. Jay will sign my discharge today."

"I hope so. I have to go now. If I don't get busy at Smithsvale, I will call you tonight."

"Take care, Michael."

"You, too."

As soon as Michael arrived at Smithsvale Hospital, he went to the ICU to visit Deanna and to see how she was doing.

He looked at the chart first. Her blood PH and blood gases were normal. She was now on Intermittent Mandatory Ventilation. Her pulmonary function tests were almost back to the level that was expected of an asthmatic. She was expected to do better and probably would soon be weaned to 40% oxygen with high humidity mask. After reading the chart, Michael went to Deanna's room and introduced himself.

"I am Michael Olsire. I am one of the doctors who took care of you yesterday. I can't believe the difference between you and the patient who came here in respiratory distress; you really look great! It is like comparing night and day."

"My parents told me all about you. We are very grateful for your kindness and concern. There are not that many doctors who would go out of their way to talk to a frightened and stressed family. There are very few doctors whose bedside manners can compare to yours. I know; I have been to several doctors for twelve years because of asthma. Unfortunately, we have this lousy HMO insurance. My father's company offers only HMO."

"The government put up this flawed healthcare policy. Tell your father that it is illegal for an employer to offer only HMO. Actually, your father and all his co-workers could take their employer to court for offering only HMO. HMO should be offered only as an option. You have a problem, though. You have a preexisting condition. I have to discuss this with your father. Please, have him page me when he comes tonight. I am so glad you are doing fine. See you later."

"Thank you, Dr. Olsire."

Michael checked the operating room schedule to see if there were patients to be seen and histories and physical examinations to be done. Most of the operating room cases were same day admissions. He went directly to his room to get some sleep.

The phone rang at seven o'clock. It was the nurse from the ICU. "Mr. Quigley wants to talk to you. He will be waiting for you in the waiting room."

"I will be there shortly."

Michael went directly to the waiting room of the ICU. Mr. and Mrs. Quigley were already waiting for him.

"Dr. Olsire, thank you for all your concern for our daughter. She told us that you are concerned about her HMO insurance."

"I am. I think you better learn more about the implications of having an HMO insurance. You have to be an assertive and informed consumer. You have to ask questions. Don't just say 'yes' to whatever the gatekeeper tells you, especially with regard to testing, referral to specialists, and admissions to hospitals. Employers are not allowed by the Federal Act of HMO 1973 to offer only HMO. HMO should only be offered as an option. You have to get together with your co-workers and convince your employer to offer commercial insurances, too. Deanna has a preexisting condition (asthma) so your employer should switch you to another insurance that would include coverage of preexisting condition in the insurance contract. It all depends on how much your employer wants to spend on healthcare benefits."

"I see. I will get together with my co-workers and the union. This way, we will have a bargaining position and alternative."

"That's a good idea."

"Thank you, Dr. Olsire."

"Call me anytime; don't hesitate to call me if you need my help. You have my address and phone number. This is the last time I will be working here. I'm just relieving for my friend."

"We are so fortunate to have met you."

"Good night, I look forward to hearing from you."

Michael went back to his call room. He tried to call Laura, but her phone was busy. So he went back to sleep.

Michael was awakened by a call from the delivery room at one o'clock in the morning.

"Dr. Olsire, please come to the delivery room immediately. We need you."

Michael ran to the labor floor. He was gasping for breath. He could not wait for the elevator.

"Where is the obstetrician?"

The nurses just looked at each other without saying any word.

"Where is the obstetrician? This patient is almost ready to push! Please call him right away."

"Dr. Olsire, this patient's obstetrician is here. He is in the doctor's room."

"I am going to get him."

"You will not be able to do it."

"Why not?"

The nurses signaled Michael to go with them around the nurses' desk.

"Dr. Dunn is spaced out. We could not wake him up. He has been sleeping for five hours now."

"Did you check his vital signs?"

"Yes, we did. We also found this empty bottle of Valium tablets by his bed. He came in drunk with a scotch bottle in his hand."

"This is terrible. Does the administration know this? How about the Director of Obstetrics?"

"They all are aware of his impairment, but everyone's eyes are closed. No one wants to make waves. His drinking problem was precipitated by a frivolous lawsuit."

"I am going to call the chief. He is accountable to the public for failing to suspend an alcoholic, drug-addicted obstetrician. I am not going to take the responsibility of delivering this baby. It's not fair to the patient or to me."

Dr. Olsire called the Chief of Obstetrics.

"I am sorry I cannot come. I don't feel good."

Michael retorted, "Dr. Bell, you'll just have to delegate your authority to another obstetrician on your staff. This is abandonment of this poor patient. She went to Dr. Dunn to be taken care of by him, not by a moonlighter who has not seen a delivery for six years. I'm going to call the administrator now, and, for your information, I have also documented this conversation on the patient's chart to protect her interests and my license. I'm not going to be part of your conspiracy of silence. Either you come now or I call the administrator."

"You are an arrogant, self-righteous man. I hope you don't have to moonlight at Smithsvale again."

"I am not arrogant. I am doing what I think is right. As far as I am concerned, the patient's welfare should come first. You are also not doing Dr. Dunn a favor by protecting him, and, at the same time, you happen to be jeopardizing his patient's life. Please come to the hospital now, you have to deliver this patient! You have to check on Dr. Dunn's mental status, too! Now!"

"I will be there as soon as I can."

Dr. Bell arrived at the delivery room ten minutes before the patient started pushing. Dr. Bell requested Michael to come with him to the doctor's room. Dr. Bell shook Dr. Dunn.

"Dr. Dunn! Dr. Dunn! Dr. Dunn!" Dr. Bell took Dr. Dunn's pulse.

"He has a weak pulse and barely audible heartbeat. Please call a code. We might be able to resuscitate him."

Dr. Bell stayed with the patient of Dr. Dunn. He introduced himself to the patient. He closed the labor room door so that the patient would not hear the commotion.

Michael helped with the code. It was too late!

The patient heard all the commotion and asked, "What's going on? How come all these doctors are rushing to the delivery room?"

"Come on, Mrs. Davis, concentrate on your pushing; you should be ready to deliver in ten minutes. Push! Push! The head is crowning out ten cents worth. We must see a quarter's worth. Then we will put up your legs. You will push better in that position."

"Thank you, Dr. Bell. You have indeed been very kind and patient. I am just sorry Dr. Dunn could not make it."

"I am sure he would not mind that I am delivering you. Just tell him the apple was ripe and it fell; the baby just could not wait for him any longer."

"I will tell him next time I see him."

"That is fine with me."

In the meantime, Michael called the administrator. Mr. Weiss immediately came to the delivery room. He waited with Michael until Dr. Bell was finished delivering Mrs. Davis. Everything went well with her delivery. She delivered an eight pound baby boy under general anaesthesia. The couple was very happy.

"Mr. Weiss, what are we going to do with Dr. Dunn's body?"

"We have to call Mrs. Dunn out of courtesy. We need to do this, though, in utmost secrecy. We can't afford any bad publicity for the medical staff and the administration. We just had a maternal death three weeks ago. Let's go down to my office, and we will call Mrs. Dunn as soon as we get there. You better tell the nurses and nurse supervisor not to tell anyone. We will make it appear that Dr. Dunn died of natural causes."

RING===RING===RING

"Good morning, Mrs. Dunn. I'm Mr. Weiss, the administrator at Smithsvale. I am sorry to bother you this early."

"That is alright. Are you looking for my husband?"

"No, I know where Dr. Dunn is. I wonder if you can come to the hospital with your station wagon?"

"Why with my station wagon?"

"We will tell you as soon as you arrive. And, please park you car near the basement garage. We will meet you there."

"I will be there in twenty minutes."

The administrator and Dr. Bell went down to the basement to meet Mrs. Dunn.

"Mrs. Dunn, we have to talk in my office," said Mr. Weiss. They all went up to the administrator's office.

"What is this all about?"

"It's about your husband. He died in his sleep in the doctor's call room. We could not awaken him when it was time for him to deliver a baby."

"Oh, my God! I knew something was not right when he left home last night. He has been so distraught since the medical malpractice suit was filed against him three months ago. It has been a nightmare for the whole family. He could not even talk to our children without screaming at them. He has been impossible to live with. If things were not going right at home, he would just scream at us. He considers being sued a personal assault to his integrity and ability as a physician. I tried to tell him that, if he had not been sued in twenty years, he would have been either a quack or not seeing enough patients. He was so unrealistic. On the day he received the summons, I found him crying in the bathroom. I could not even hold his hand. He was in a lot of emotional pain. He also had several nightmares. Sometimes, he would wake up screaming and sweating. The stress and emotional pain my husband experienced are similar to what veterans experienced in the Post-Vietnam Stress Syndrome. Doctors need to establish a national network for their colleagues who are experiencing stress, depression, and emotional turmoil because of the trauma of medical malpractice suits. I don't mean to imply that medical doctors don't commit medical malpractice, but lawyers should differentiate between maloccurrence and blatant medical negligence. In the city of Philadelphia, there are too many unethical lawyers. The city is saturated with 14,000 lawyers. We have more lawyers in this city than there are in Japan."

"Mrs. Dunn, Dr. Bell and I fully understand what you are trying to say. The whole society is at fault."

"But my husband did not do anything to hurt the patient who sued him! He scheduled her for testing, and she canceled! Then she became sick later and developed complications; she had the gall to blame and sue my husband for her own lack of responsibility! Where is justice?"

"Mrs. Dunn, there is so much injustice that we see in the legal system, but the legal profession is too powerful. Two-thirds of the members of Congress are lawyers. Why would they legislate against themselves? We cannot even get a tort reform in Pennsylvania; politicians, however, want us to give free care."

"I know. I am so devastated. This unethical lawyer has destroyed our lives."

"What is this shark's name?"

"His name is Robert Smith. The day will come when someone will go after him for revenge, and I will be one of those seeking retribution."

"We are with you all the way, Mrs. Dunn. You know, he might sue your husband's estate and make the estate the defendant."

"I have the gut feeling he will continue the suit until he is able to milk money from the insurance company and from me."

"Now, let's go up. Mrs. Dunn, please wash your face. I will get you a cup of coffee. Mrs. Dunn, we really should not let anyone know the full circumstances surrounding your husband's death. Robert Smith might be able to use it to prove your husband's impairment and incompetence. We think it would be better for you to take him home and say that he died in his sleep there."

"Thank you for your kindness, both of you."

Mrs. Dunn, Dr. Bell, and the administrator tiptoed through the exit doors until they reached the delivery room. They went inside the doctor's room where the body of Dr. Dunn was kept wrapped with white linen sheets. Dr. Bell unwrapped the body so that Mrs. Dunn could view her husband. She kissed his forehead and then started sobbing, "Ryan, how could you do this to us? What will I tell the children?"

"Mrs. Dunn, do you want to call your children?"

"No, I want to take his body home first."

"We will go with you. Dr. Bell will drive your husband's car, and I will drive your station wagon. I will drive the station wagon inside the garage, and we will have to carry the body into your bedroom. We can wake up the kids after we have unwrapped Ryan's body."

"Thank you for your understanding. I don't know what I would have done without your help. It would have been traumatic for the kids to see this in the newspaper or hear it on the radio or see it on television."

In the meantime, Michael stayed in the doctor's room and tried to straighten up. He felt so sad for Mrs. Dunn. It had been a harrowing experience for her.

Michael went back to his room exhausted and unable to sleep. He could still see the anguished face of the dead man.

"Dr. Ryan Dunn gave up to an unfair legal system when he started drinking and taking drugs to lessen his emotional pain and suffering. The inequitable legal system has taken its toll on the medical establishment."

CHAPTER XV

Michael woke up at seven in the morning. This was quite late for him; he had been busy between four and five with calls from the ICU. He took a quick shower and passed by the cafeteria for a cup of coffee.

Laura was already dressed when he arrived at Northend Hospital.

"It is almost nine-thirty. We will still be able to catch the ten o'clock mass for Charlie at Miraculous Medal Church."

"Is Charlie going to be cremated?"

"I think so."

The church was barely filled when they arrived. Patty was sitting in the front pew with Mrs. Collins, Kathy, and Michelle.

When the mass was over, Michael and Laura waited near the church entrance for the bereaved family. Michael and Laura extended their condolences.

"Please don't hesitate to call us if there is anything we can do to help."

"Charlie is going to be cremated. We're going to ask for the ashes so that we can keep them at home. Thank you for coming to the mass and for all your support. We will never be able to repay you for all the time you spent visiting and talking to Charlie."

"I know this Christmas will be a difficult one for you, but we will be thinking of all of you. I know it might sound odd, but I want to wish you a peaceful and happy holiday."

"Thank you," Patty sobbed. "This could have been a very happy Christmas for us; it was not meant to be. I just hope Charlie is at peace and that Geoffrey is living with a nice and lovely couple."

"Patty, I assure you that Geoffrey is in good hands."

"Thank you."

Michael and Laura hugged everyone and left.

"Michael, may we pass by the mall?"

"You might get dizzy. It is a pretty big mall to walk around."

"We will just walk around the jewelry stores. I just want to see some jewelry for Mom and Jeanie."

"It will be alright then. Are you hungry?"

"No, I ate my breakfast at the hospital. How about you?"

"I only had a cup of coffee. I was up all night. It was a nightmare. Dr. Ryan Dunn died in the doctor's room in the delivery room."

"He was a nice and conscientious obstetrician."

"Had you met him?"

"Yes, I have assisted him on two Caesarean sections. What happened? Why did he die in the delivery room?"

"We don't really know. He became depressed three months ago after he was sued frivolously by a lawyer named Robert Smith."

"That name sounds familiar. Isn't that the Robert Smith who messed up Charlie?"

"Yes, but there are many lawyers in Philadelphia named Robert Smith. We have no idea if this Robert Smith is the same Robert Smith who deals in drugs, using homeless people like Charlie."

"We have to find out then."

"How?"

"We have to stay with Charlie's friends downtown to see if Robert Smith comes around with his fifty cc syringe filled with cocaine."

"We can't do that."

"Why not?"

"Five of Charlie's fellow homeless are all in University Hospital, felled by AIDS. I don't know how many more homeless in Charlie's group are left on the streets."

"This lawyer is getting away with it, though!"

"I know."

"This is so sad. It's as tragic as the case of the lady who died three weeks ago at Smithsvale Hospital. She bled to death because the insurance company wouldn't let her stay in the hospital until she delivered. She was discharged on bedrest at home even though she was spotting every time she moved. The obstetrician, the insurance company, the nurse, and the doctor utilization reviewer should all be sued for medical negligence, conspiracy, and racketeering. It would have made a lot of difference if the patient had been in the hospital, but no one saw it that way. Only the bottom line and their pocketbooks mattered to them."

"Laura, how can you talk like that?"

"Because I am very upset that Mrs. Dunn lost her husband because of the greedy lawyer who sued Dr. Dunn frivolously. Mrs. Dunn did not only lose her husband, she was also robbed of herself. She was robbed of her identity. Her life will never be the same."

"Robert Smith should be sued for abuse of the legal system and hedonic damage after Mrs. Dunn's lawyer gets this frivolous case thrown out of court."

"I was so upset when that lady bled to death that I cried. The obstetrician did not care. All he wanted to do was to write up the chart to protect himself. All he said to the shocked and grieving widower was a terse, 'I'm sorry, your wife did not make it'! I overheard him. He did not even bother sitting down with the husband and explaining to the poor man why his wife bled to death. How about this poor patient who died needlessly because she fell through the cracks of cost-containment? How about the husband and the child whose lives have been ruined? How about the husband and the child whose vision of the future has been replaced by uncertainty and a dark cloud? How about the husband who lost his best friend, lover, and companion? How about the baby who will never know, feel and experience the warmth, love, and tenderness of a nurturing mother? I know money will never ease the pain, grief, and suffering of the family. Money will not bring her back, but the only way to get back at greedy and uncaring physicians is through their pocketbooks."

"Laura, you are getting upset about situations you can't control."

"I am getting disillusioned with organized medicine. It is mostly our fault that patients are suffering. We have let the government and all the healthcare insurance companies take over the practice of medicine. We deserve what we are getting from everyone. When is the medical profession going to stand up to protect the interest of patients? When is the medical profession going to stand up against the government's and healthcare insurance companies' interference?"

"Laura, I did not realize you were a radical."

"I am not a radical. I care."

"I care, too, but at least I am realistic. We need numbers. There is power in numbers."

"I know, but these gutless doctors will not do anything until they are hit in their pocketbooks."

"I know; you don't need to tell me that. It is so obvious. Here we are. We can't walk too long."

"Yes, doctor. I thought you wanted to get something to eat first!"

"Okay. Let's go and get something to eat first."

"That would be fine."
"Do you want to eat lunch or brunch?"
"Just something light should be fine. We can both have lunch at home."
Laura and Michael had coffee and danish. After they finished eating, they went to a jewelry store.
Laura's eyes sparkled when she saw a sapphire cocktail ring surrounded by small diamonds. She saw two gold necklaces that she wanted to buy for her mom and Jeanie. She had them daintily Christmas gift-wrapped. Michael was silently watching Laura.
Michael and Laura arrived at 90064 Kalina St. at one in the afternoon. Mrs. Secula and Jeanie were both decorating the Christmas tree.
"Are you two going to have lunch first before you help decorating the Christmas tree?"
"Mom, don't worry, I will prepare our lunch. Michael can help with the decorations while I work in the kitchen."
"We have some lasagna, spaghetti, and chicken left-over from last night. Probably, Michael would rather have that than a sandwich."
"What do you say, Michael?"
"I think I like that idea. I would rather eat something hot."
"I will heat them all then. Michael, do you want wine, too?"
"I think so."
"It will take only ten minutes."
Ten minutes later, Laura walked into the living room.
"Michael, lunch is ready."
"I will be there. Thank you." Michael sat down at the table and started eating.
"This is really good. What is the Italian name for this dish?"
"Chicken Cacciatore. Mom has been very conscious of what we eat since Dad died of a massive heart attack. We are not allowed to eat butter and junk food."
"I can understand that. Don't you want to go to a second-hand car dealer today?"
"Only for a couple of hours. I just want to choose the car today and then apply for a loan at the bank Tuesday."
"I think that is a good idea. It would save time."
"Why don't you take me to the car dealer in Bustleton? I would like to get a Chevy."
"That is a good idea. We better patronize our own products; otherwise, we will lose the economic war to Japan."
"I agree with you. What do you want for dessert?"
"I am pretty full. I will pass."
"Let us get going then. I know you are tired. Just drop me off after we are done doing business at the car dealer. You have to get some sleep."
"Thank you for caring."
The manager at the used car lot was very pleasant and helpful. Laura was hoping to find a navy blue Chevy.
"When are you going to pick this up?"
"I have to apply for a car loan first."
"We have a car loan financing department, and the rates are competitive with the commercial banks."
"When would I know that my loan is approved?"
"I can check your credit rating now."
"I don't really have any credit cards. I am only a resident. Who would give me credit cards when I am not even making much money?"

"It does not matter. You have a good earning potential as all doctors do. Why don't you look over our used car lot while I am doing a credit check on you? You should be able to pick up the car by December 26th after twelve noon. All the necessary papers will be ready for your signature."

"Thank you."

Michael and Laura went over about ten used Chevy cars.

"I think I will take the blue, four-door Chevy sedan."

"That car is in good shape. Why don't you try driving it first?"

"I will ask the salesman for the keys."

Laura drove the car. The car ran smoothly without any noise or hesitation.

"Michael, this car is just right for me."

"I am glad. Let us tell the salesman so that he can put a sold tag on it."

They went back to the office.

"I have chosen the blue, four-door Chevy sedan."

"You can pick it up on December 26th. You have good credit rating. All the papers will be ready for your signature when you come in."

"Thank you, and Merry Christmas."

"Laura, I will just drop you off. I have to pick up something at the mall."

"Can I go with you?"

"No, you need to rest, just like your patients need to rest after they are discharged from the hospital."

"I know. Are you in a hurry to get home?"

"Yes. I want to get some sleep. Did you get today's paper?"

"No."

"Well, I will get one at the mall. I want to see if the obituary section will have Dr. Dunn's death notice."

"Tomorrow's paper will probably have it."

"We are here now. I hope you don't mind if I don't go up to say hello to your Mom and Jeanie. Please explain to them I am in a hurry."

"I will do that."

Michael went back to the jewelry store at the mall. He looked at the display counters where he had seen Laura looking at the sapphire cocktail ring.

"May I see that sapphire cocktail ring, please? What size is it?"

"Size 6 1/2."

"I would like to put down a deposit on it. Will you be open Christmas Eve?"

"Yes, we will be open until midnight."

"Could you please wrap it for me? I will pick it up in the afternoon."

"It will be ready when you come."

Michael could not find the evening edition of the *Philadelphia Gazette* at the mall.

"I hope I find one in the hospital."

It took Michael over an hour to get back from the mall. Traffic was really heavy; people were trying to finish their last minute Christmas shopping. He also witnessed a head-on collision on the expressway. The victims were all rushed to the accident wards of nearby hospitals.

Michael dropped by the hospital to see if there was a *Philadelphia Gazette* left at the newsstand. He found one and looked over the obituary section which read:

Dr. Ryan Dunn, a graduate of Dorchester Medical School, died in his sleep at home.

He is survived by his wife, Marguerite, and two sons, Ryan Jr. and Brian. Viewing and mass at 9:00 a.m. at our Lady of Perpetual Help in Montgomery County. Donations to the American Cancer Society will be appreciated by the family.

Michael called Laura. "I found the obituary of Dr. Dunn. Do you want to attend the mass? I will pick you up at eight in the morning. The viewing will be in Montgomery County."

"You better get some sleep then. I know you are tired. Good night. See you in the morning."

At exactly eight in the morning, Michael was at the Secula driveway. Laura was ready, also.

"I feel so sorry for Mrs. Dunn and the boys. They were a nice couple. One night I was on call when she came in with her two boys; they were quite a family. I heard he had Hodgkin's Disease, too, and was in remission; this frivolous suit filed by Robert Smith really depressed him. That lawyer should be disbarred. I hope Mrs. Dunn will go after him when the case is dismissed. The only way to fight greedy lawyers is to hurt them where it will hurt most, their pocketbooks."

"I agree with you. It works both ways. This theory applies to greedy doctors, too. Their medical judgement is usually clouded by the color of the dollar."

"Greedy doctors and greedy lawyers both deserve to be sued and to be made accountable for their actions."

"You can't do it, though."

"Why not?"

"Conspiracy of silence protects them."

"Since we are both disillusioned by what we see in the medical and legal professions, why don't we become J.D.'s?"

"It would be like going from construction to demolition."

"But there are good and bad apples in all professions."

"But I think medicine is better; it is a helping profession. There is more human interaction, and the psychological dividend that a doctor experiences is very emotionally satisfying and priceless."

"I agree with you."

"This must be Perpetual Help Church. It is crowded."

"Dr. Dunn was very well-liked by his colleagues."

"That is understandable."

"Come on, the line is quite long. We have to meet the family."

Laura introduced herself to Mrs. Dunn and hugged her.

"Dr. Secula, my husband mentioned your name to me a couple of times. He was very impressed with your compassion for patients."

"Thank you, Mrs. Dunn."

"Dr. Olsire, it's so nice of you to come. Thank you for all your kindness and for covering for my husband that morning."

"You are welcome, Mrs. Dunn. I wish I could have done more."

After all the people had conveyed their condolences to Mrs. Dunn, mass started. There were about 500 people inside the church. The eulogy was given by Ryan Jr.. He broke down before he could finish what he wanted to say. Everyone was teary-eyed and grief-stricken. Practically everyone received communion.

Laura and Michael stayed until the funeral cortege left.

"Why don't we get something to eat and then go back to the mall? Do you think you will be up to it?"

"I think so. I am strong enough to walk in the mall the whole afternoon."

After lunch, they went back to the mall. The mall was crowded. There was hardly a store where people were not standing in line at the cash registers to pay for merchandise. Santa Claus was busy posing for pictures with children in their X'mas outfits.

"Michael, let us sit for a while. The store where we are supposed to go is too crowded."

"How about waiting for me here? I'm going to join the line now so we can save time. You can stay here and watch the Christmas carolers or Santa Claus with the children. Do you want me to get you something first?"

"No, I will be fine. I should have brought something to read."

"That's alright. Just rest and relax."

Michael was the twentieth person in line. The line was hardly moving because practically every customer was using a credit card.

Michael had to wait for one and half hours before the salesperson was ready for him. The ring was already wrapped. The salesperson handed Michael a warranty. Michael paid in cash, and the salesperson gave him a receipt.

It was already four o'clock by the time they got back to the Secula residence.

"Do you want a cup of coffee?"

"I will have one. I have to get back to the hospital by five o'clock. I have to recheck one post-operative patient."

"Are you not going to join us for our Christmas Eve celebration and midnight mass?"

"I will be back later. I will see you then."

After Michael left, Laura asked Jeanie to take her to the mall.

"Why didn't you buy the present while you were at the mall?"

"I did not want Michael to see it."

"Let's go before the mall gets too crowded."

"We are not staying that long. I am only buying one item."

By the time Jeanie and Laura arrived at the mall, the mall was jammed. People were hardly moving. Christmas carols were in full blast. Children were thrilled to see Santa and have their pictures taken on his lap.

Finally, Laura decided to go to an exclusive men's store. She bought a striped silk tie for Michael and had it gift-wrapped.

"That was quick."

"I had seen this tie yesterday, but I did not want Michael to see it. I have never seen him wear the color or style of this necktie."

"It is nice and stylish."

Mrs. Secula was still in the kitchen baking cookies when Laura and Jeanie arrived.

"I have a sneaking suspicion that Michael is up to something."

"Like what, Mom?"

"I think he is going to ask you to marry him."

"Mom, Michael and I are just good friends."

"I know that, but I think you are both lovestruck. It is so obvious when you look at each other. Sometimes, both of you forget that Jeanie and I are also around the dinner table with you. There is so much chemistry between the two of you."

"Mom, my relationship with Michael is purely platonic. We communicate very well; we believe in the same ideals, and we can discuss anything without fear of being ridiculed or betrayed. We make each other feel very comfortable. We are soulmates. We care very deeply about each other, but most of all we have a lot of respect for each other. He respects me as a person and as a doctor."

"I am glad to hear that. He seems so serious when he talks."

"I know. Michael has been through a lot. Remember, he was orphaned by a drunken driver. He grew up knowing only one relative, his uncle, Father John."

"He is a nice man. He would be good for you. I think you really complement each other."

"Mom, are you trying to marry me off?"

"Laura, you are of age. If you told me you wanted to marry Michael tomorrow, I would be thrilled to gain a very nice son-in-law."

"We have to get dinner ready. Michael should be coming back soon."

"What time did you tell him to come?"

"Seven o'clock."

It was almost seven-twenty, and Michael had not arrived yet. The phone rang.

"Laura, this is Michael. I am sorry, but I do not think I will be able to make it tonight. There was a big accident on Walnut Street. Four seriously injured Septa passengers are being prepped for surgery. I have to help one of the residents. I promise I will be there tomorrow. I hope you understand."

"I understand, Michael. I will see you tomorrow."

"Laura, I will call you as soon as we are finished in the operating room. May I call you even if it is after 11:30 tonight?"

"You can call me anytime."

It was almost seven in the morning when Laura woke up. Michael had not called back. She called the university hospital. The operator said that Michael had been operating the whole night. Laura hung up. "I hope the patient made it; I hope he does well."

By nine in the morning, the operation was finally over. Michael called Laura. "We just finished the operation. We had to do splenectomy and bowel resection on an unprepared bowel. I hope the patient makes it and does not develop an infection."

"I hope so, too."

"I have to go to the church on Chestnut St. I will see you tonight."

"Be careful driving, Michael. I know you must be very tired. You have not had any sleep at all. Please get some sleep before you come down. We will be waiting for you. Merry Christmas."

"Merry Christmas to you, too. Would you please wake me up at five o'clock? Thank you."

"I will do that."

By seven o'clock, Michael was already at the Secula residence. The house was well decorated with Christmas trimmings. A nativity scene was under a live, six-foot Christmas tree. Michael placed his presents for the Secula family underneath the Christmas tree. Laura was watching him closely. She noticed that Michael kept a small gift-wrapped box inside his suit pocket. She was looking at his pocket with curiosity. Michael noticed her and asked, "What's wrong, Laura?"

"Nothing. Let's go to the dining room so I can get you a glass of eggnog. Mom, Michael is here now."

"Merry Christmas, Michael." Mrs. Secula approached Michael and hugged him. Laura was smiling as she watched the interaction between her mom and Michael.

Jeanie walked in all dressed up with her friends from work.

"Merry Christmas to everyone," greeted Mrs. Secula.

"Merry Christmas, Mrs. Secula."

"Can I get you something to drink?"

"Mrs. Secula, don't worry about us. We will help ourselves."

"Dinner will be ready by eight o'clock. There are some Christmas cookies in the living room. Help yourselves."

Mrs. Secula, Jeanie, and Laura were busy fixing and arranging the dining table and the sitting arrangements. Everything looked so perfect - the exquisite bone china, the silver, and the Christmas flower arrangement. Mrs. Secula was a regular party giver before her husband became ill. She enjoyed gourmet cooking.

Everyone sat down for dinner by eight o'clock. Mrs. Secula's crown roast was a big hit. Everyone asked for seconds. Dessert was a homemade Italian Rum Cake, some pastries, and tortes. The conversation was lively and sometimes downright funny. By nine-thirty, dinner was done. Jeanie took her guests into the living room where they sang Christmas songs. Laura helped her mom clear the table and clean up. Michael stayed with them in the kitchen.

"Michael, you are deep in thought and restless; what's wrong?"

"Nothing, Mrs. Secula, I'm just thinking of my uncle who raised me, Father John. I did not have a chance to talk to him. Everytime I called, he was not in the convent. He was either visiting sick parishioners in the hospital or saying a mass."

"Well, you can call him from here."

"I will call him later. Laura can talk to him, too."

Laura was perplexed.

By ten-thirty, Jeanie's guests were getting ready to leave. Michael gave a sigh of relief.

Michael wanted to talk to Mrs. Secula first. Mrs. Secula took Michael by the hand to the kitchen.

"Michael, what can I do for you? You look so serious."

"Mrs. Secula, I want to ask your permission to marry Laura."

"Have you asked her yet?"

"Not yet."

"Well, as far as I am concerned, you can marry Laura anytime. But you must ask her first. I would love to have you as my son-in-law. You are a very nice man."

Mrs. Secula called Laura to the kitchen.

"Laura, Michael wants to tell you something."

Michael pulled out the small gift-wrapped box from his pocket and gave it to Laura.

Laura immediately opened the box. She got so excited! "Michael, this is the same cocktail sapphire ring I was admiring at the jewelry store! You must have been watching me closely while we were there!"

Michael took the ring from Laura and put it onto her left ring finger and asked, "Laura, would you marry me?"

Laura could not control her emotions any longer. She hugged and kissed Michael. "I thought you would not ask me again."

Michael replied, "I can take 'no' for an answer the first time, but not the second time. Would you marry me on St. Patty's Day?"

"Yes, I will."

Mrs. Secula and Jeanie were watching the two lovebirds. Mrs. Secula cried with happiness.

"Thank God, my daughter's found a good man!"

Jeanie said, "I would love to be the maid of honor!"

"Naturally, you are my only sister. We have to start shopping for our outfits; we don't have that much time left."

"Laura, let's call Father John and ask him if he can come and officiate at our wedding."

"That's a good idea."

Michael dialed the phone. Father John answered after three rings.

"Merry Christmas, Father John."

"Merry Christmas, Michael. How have you been? We were just talking about you. I saw the dean from the medical school yesterday. He asked me how you were doing. How is everything?"

"Father, I am doing well. I have good news to tell you. I'm getting married on St. Patty's day. I want you to talk to my fiancee, Laura. I will put her on."

"How are you, Father John? I know all about you. Michael has told me all the good things you did for him. Thank you for raising such a nice man for me. Would you be able to officiate at our wedding? We would like you to come one week early so that we would have time to get acquainted. I would love you to meet my mother and sister, too. My father died almost a year ago. Michael and I met at the emergency room the night we brought my father there. It is ironic how such a misfortune turned out to be so fortuitous. It was really God's will that I meet Michael. I hope you will be able to bless our marriage."

"Laura, I am going to be there one week before the wedding as you've requested. Michael has told me a lot of things about you as well! I feel that this is a love match made in heaven. You really complement each other in many ways. I know you will both be very happy. You are both mature and idealistic. Please, let me talk to Michael."

After Laura gave the phone to Michael, Father John said, "Michael, would you like Laura to have some of your scrapbooks?"

"I know she will be thrilled to see them. I am making one for her, too. I was hoping to be able to give it to her as a Christmas gift, but too many things came up. I am going to give it to her on Valentine's Day instead. It is two hundred pages. I have about ten pages left to fill with dried flowers. I should be able to finish it in two weeks. Father John, I will call you again this week. Also, could you please get me the phone number of my godfather? I would like him and his wife to come to our wedding."

"I will have it ready for you when you call. Good night, Michael. You and Laura have a Happy New Year!"

"Good night, Father John."

After Michael got off the phone, he said to Laura, "It's almost twelve midnight. I better go home. I will pick you up tomorrow so that you can get your car."

"Good night, Michael. Call me before you come."

"Good night, Mrs. Secula and Jeanie."

"Good night, Michael. Be careful driving. It is starting to snow now."

After Michael left, Laura turned on the television to check the weather report. Small snowflakes were falling. Driving was treacherous. The temperature was only twenty-nine degrees. Laura looked out the window to see if Michael was still there, but Michael's car was already gone.

Later, Laura tossed in bed. It was already two-thirty in the morning. She was debating whether to call Michael to see how he made out with the treacherous driving. She stood up and looked out the window. All of Kalina Street was covered with almost four inches of snow. Finally, she decided to call Michael. The phone rang twelve times before Michael answered.

"Michael, did I wake you up?"

"No, I just arrived. Driving was treacherous. The roads were icy and slippery. Traffic was not moving on the Schuylkill Expressway. There were three accidents on the expressway alone. I am fine. I was going to call you, but you beat me to it. I know I must have worried you to death!"

"I am just glad you are fine. I will be able to sleep now. Good night, Michael. I will see you tomorrow."

"Good night, Laura, and thank you for caring."

CHAPTER XVI

Laura was still off from work. She had to wait until December 28th before her doctor would let her go back.

By twelve noon, the city workers had finished plowing the main streets. Michael called Laura.

"I am tied up. A heavyset man walked into the emergency room with ruptured aneurysm. We are just pumping blood, and we'll be taking him to the operating room shortly. I don't know how long this surgery will last. The guy is only 35-years-old, but he is a little on the heavy side."

"Do whatever you have to do. Jeanie can take me tonight if your surgery lasts that long. I hope this poor man makes it."

"I hope so, too."

It was already six o'clock in the evening, and still Michael had not called. Laura called the university hospital. Michael was still in the operating room.

Laura decided to have Jeanie drive her to the used car lot. By the time they arrived at the car dealer's office, all the paper work was ready. All that was needed was Laura's signature. Laura and Jeanie went over the contract before Laura signed it. The car was ready to go. It was polished inside and out and was shiny.

Laura drove very slowly. The small streets which were not plowed were very icy. Laura followed Jeanie's route. Laura's car stalled and she could not start it. Jeanie stopped to see how Laura was doing. The motor died and would not restart. Finally, Laura and Jeanie decided to leave the car and go home. It was almost ten o'clock when they reached home. The phone was ringing. Mrs. Secula had fallen asleep on the sofa. Laura ran towards the phone. It was Michael calling. "I've just finished the operation. The patient is doing better and is being monitored in the ICU."

"I am glad."

"Were you able to pick up your car?"

"Yes and no."

"What do you mean?"

"Well, Jeanie and I picked up the car. It looked nice and well-polished. But, we were halfway between the car dealer and our house when it stopped running. I could not get it started."

"Do you want me to come down now to see if we can get it started?"

"No, you are too tired and sleepy. I will call the car dealer tomorrow."

"Let me know how you make out. I will call you between operating room cases. Are you going back to work Wednesday?"

"Yes, if I can get this car fixed. I'm supposed to start moonlighting at Southern Hospital."

"What department are you going to moonlight in?"

"The emergency room. I don't want to work on the floors anymore. I get very upset when I see all the lonely, elderly patients. It is very depressing. They do not get the nursing care they need because of the shortage of nurses. Sometimes they don't even have relatives to visit them or any place to go home to; the nursing homes won't take them because they have no money or insurance. It's such a vicious cycle."

"Laura, you can't solve the problems of the world. But I am glad you are aware of what's going on."

"Don't politicians realize how flawed their healthcare policies are?"

"I don't know; I am beginning to think they just don't care. They have Bethesda Hospital and the helicopters to fly them to Bethesda courtesy of the poor taxpayers."

"I think politicians should not stay too long in office. They should be limited to two terms."

"I think so, too. But who are we to say that? We don't have any money or political clout. Our opinions probably don't count either."

"I will probably see you tomorrow."

"Good night."

Laura woke up early. She tried to call the car dealer at 8:00 a.m., but there was no answer. Jeanie drove Laura to the place where they left the car. It was nowhere to be found. Laura called the police department in the neighborhood. The car had been towed; she would have to shell out $150.00 to get it back.

Finally, Laura was able to get in touch with the car dealer.

"My car stalled last night on Byberry Road. We could not get it restarted. You were already closed at that time. So, we left it in the street. I just called the police department, and the officer at the desk told me it had to be towed. The car was a public hazard since it was parked in the middle of an icy road. I think you are responsible for getting it back to your lot and getting it fixed."

"I don't think so. Once you got the keys of the car and drove it out of the parking lot, the responsibility was all yours."

"But you sold me a defective car!"

"It was running when you drove it out of the lot."

"I know, but the alternator and the batteries were in bad shape."

"I can't do anything about that. You can have the car towed back to the lot, and we'll try to fix it at no charge to you. That's the best deal we can give you."

"I will call the towing company. I would like to pick it up tonight."

"No problem."

Laura was quite upset. Now she really had to get extra night calls not only to save money for the wedding, but also to pay off the car.

Michael called at twelve noon.

"Laura, how are you doing? Did you get your car fixed yet?"

"Not yet."

"I will give you a call later. I have to scrub for the next case. Talk to you soon."

"Don't work too hard."

Laura got a call from the car dealer.

"We have to change the alternator. It will cost $350.00 plus labor."

"I don't think I should pay for it. You sold me a second-hand lemon. I have to report you to the business bureau. You are trying to take advantage of me. This is the end of it. I would like to talk to the president of your company."

"I will connect you to him now. His name is Mr. Stone."

Laura waited patiently for Mr. Stone to answer the phone.

"Mr. Stone, I am very dissatisfied with the transaction I had with your company. I bought a second-hand lemon which is not running at all. I can't afford to buy a new alternator. The second-hand car I bought from you stalled as soon as I got out of your lot. This is a terrible business practice. I am going to return that car and not pay my monthly installment if I have to shell out $350.00."

"Dr. Secula, don't worry about the $350.00. I will take care of your alternator. You can pick up the car at five o'clock today."

"Thank you very much, sir. I really appreciate your goodwill and understanding. I will try to be there before you close at nine o'clock."

"If there is any way we can be of service, just give us a call."

"Thank you."

Michael was on the phone at exactly five o'clock.

"Laura, I am just waiting for the traffic to ease off. I should be there by seven o'clock."

"You can have dinner with us."

"Thank you, but I had dinner ten minutes ago."

Laura sat down with her Mom and Jeanie. They were discussing the bridal outfit.

"I am going to wear a white satin gown with a high Victorian neckline and flared skirt. The skirt will have applique at the center decorated with mini white roses, and I am going to carry a bouquet of gardenias."

"I would like to wear a long pink empire gown. I am going to carry a white rose bouquet with a matching headdress."

"I have chosen a long blue gown with a matching handbag."

"We better do our trousseau shopping this week. We have only two months and twenty-one days left. I have called several restaurants and most of them are already booked. The three Italian restaurants that are not yet booked are Fabiola, Genova, and Sorrento. You and Michael can discuss this tonight after you get your car from the dealer."

"We can also make our guest list and decide where to order the invitations and flowers. Michael and I have decided that we would both foot the wedding bill."

"That's very thoughtful of Michael."

By seven o'clock, Michael was pulling into the Secula driveway. He came up and said hello to everyone.

"Michael, we have to get going. We have a lot of things to talk about. We have to decide where we will hold the reception. We can go to church tonight and talk to the pastor to see if he will let Father John officiate at our wedding ceremony."

"Why don't you call the pastor now to see if he has time to see us before we pick up your car?"

Laura called up Father Walls.

"I will be glad to talk to both of you."

Laura and Michael rushed to St. Archangel's Church. Father Walls was already at the sacristy waiting for them.

"I know both of you are good practicing Catholics, but you still have to attend the Pre-Canaan Conference once a week for six weeks. If there is any conflict with your busy schedule, please let me know."

Michael said, "We will try to adjust our schedule according to the parish schedule. This class is very important to both of us."

"I will see you at the Pre-Canaan Conference."

"Thank you for seeing us tonight, Father."

"Take care, both of you."

Laura and Michael rushed to the car dealer. It was almost eight-thirty in the evening. They barely made it. Laura signed all the papers, and the manager gave her the keys to the car.

"Sorry for the inconvenience. I hope this car runs well for you."

"I hope so, too."

Laura drove first and Michael followed her. They reached the Secula residence without the car stalling again.

"Michael, do you want a cup of coffee?"

"No, thank you."

"Now we have to decide on our guest list."

"Here are the only guests I want to invite: Dr. Jay Simmons, his daughter, Debbie, Jorge and Estela, John Miller and his wife, James Dillon and his wife, my godfather and his wife, and my six residents. The rest of the guests will be your family. I don't even have cousins because my father and mother were both only children. You have enough relatives in South Philadelphia to make up the one hundred guests we intend to invite."

"Here is a note from Mom that Sorrento can accommodate one hundred guests. It is still available for March 17th."

"We should call Sorrento tomorrow."

"We can even go there tomorrow after work."

"Why don't you make an appointment for seven o'clock?"

"I will meet you here at six o'clock. You can have dinner with us."

Laura's eyes were caught by the headline in the newspaper which Michael had brought: "Three bodies recovered from Schuylkill believed to be patients of Perseverance Mental Hospital."

The three bodies had been retrieved from the icy Schuylkill River. These three patients had been missing from the hospital grounds for two weeks now. The families of the victims had been notified. The medical examiner's report would be released in two weeks. There was no evidence of foul play. The patients had died from accidental drowning.

"This is asinine! How could three patients from a mental institution reach the Schuylkill without any transportation? Is there no security at this institution?"

"I don't know. This is a very sad situation. The mentally ill deserve better treatment from society. The healthcare system for the mentally ill is on the verge of collapse. Politicians don't care. We must find a better way to treat this type of patient."

"In the local newspaper, I just read a letter written by a friend of a depressed patient. This patient committed suicide after he had been denied admission to a mental hospital because he had no healthcare insurance. This is just unconscionable. A patient requested help; he knew he was suicidal. The hospital denied him that help; he went home and killed himself."

"How tragic."

"This is the type of patient who is denied care most of the time. Most healthcare insurances pay only up to thirty days for psychiatric care; then the patient is switched to Medicaid. The reimbursement from Medicaid is so low that the hospitals would rather admit paying patients."

"It is a shame. This is the worst disease that you can have because you have no control. A mentally ill patient becomes dependent on drugs which sometimes don't even work; the patient ends up becoming worse rather than better."

"I could not agree more."

"The whole healthcare system needs a complete overhaul."

"It is getting late now. I will see you tomorrow at six o'clock."

CHAPTER XVII

Laura was not home when Michael pulled into the Secula residence. Mrs. Secula answered the doorbell.

"Come in, Michael. Laura is going to be thirty minutes late. Her last surgical case was delayed. The patient had some abnormal laboratory tests, and they had to be repeated."

"Mrs. Secula, you don't have to explain anything. I understand; I have stood up Laura many times because of my operating room schedule."

"I will prepare dinner for you then."

"I can wait for Laura. We can have dinner together. Please, don't wait for us."

"I have eaten dinner already. Jeanie had to visit her friend in the hospital. We ate at five o'clock. We can watch the evening news while we are waiting for her. Which channel do you want to watch?"

"No channel in particular. It is up to you."

Laura pulled into the driveway. She ran in and kissed her mom. "We have to get going. We can eat later when we come back from Sorrento. The manager will only be there until eight o'clock. The room available is upstairs and is good for only 110 people. This is the only restaurant available for our March 17th date. We better hurry up."

"Laura, you are out of breath and tired. You better drink orange juice or eat something; you might pass out. You must be hungry since you were in the operating room the whole day. I bet you did not have time to eat."

"You are really a mind reader, Michael. I will bring a small can of orange juice and some cookies. I will eat in the car."

"That's fine with me."

Mr. Benza, the manager of Sorrento restaurant and hotel, was waiting for them when they arrived.

"Would you like a drink, or, perhaps, you would like to try our menu?"

Trying to signal him to say 'yes,' Laura looked at Michael.

"Do you have filet mignon or roast beef?"

"Yes, we do. Would you like to try them both and then decide which one you want for your wedding? We also have some dessert available."

"That will be nice."

Laura and Michael sat down and tried each of the meats and the dessert.

"Laura, what do you think?"

"I think the tender roast beef wins my vote. How about you, Michael?"

"I agree with you."

"The strawberry shortcake and parfait would be perfect."

"I think so, too."

"Are you going to have an open bar?"

"Only for two hours. I don't want anything to happen to any of our guests on their way home. I want everyone to leave the reception sober for the drive home."

"That is very thoughtful of you."

Michael and Laura discussed the table arrangement, menu, open bar, and flower arrangements with Mr. Benza. They signed the contract and left.

It was almost eleven o'clock when they pulled into the Secula driveway.

"Laura, I can't stay. I have to be home early. We have another grand round tomorrow. We also have to look for an apartment tomorrow, midway between our hospitals."

"Why don't you pick me up at the hospital? We will have dinner at Northend Hospital, and afterwards we will look for an apartment."

"I will try to be at Northend Hospital by five o'clock."

"Michael, please call first. Our operating room schedule tomorrow is really busy."

"I will do that."

Michael gave Laura a good night kiss.

"Be careful driving. Call me when you get home."

"Okay, Laura."

The next day, Michael called Laura. She was still tied up in the operating room at five o'clock.

As soon as Laura was finished, she called Michael.

"Michael, can you be here by six o'clock?"

"Yes, I was just waiting for your call. I will be there shortly."

As soon as Michael pulled into the emergency room parking lot, he saw Laura waving at him.

"I've got two sandwiches and a couple of cans of diet Pepsi for us. I called Jelton Realty, and the manager will wait for us until eight o'clock."

"We should be there by seven o'clock. We will have time to see several apartments."

Mr. Jelton, the owner's son, greeted them in the lobby. Laura and Michael decided to rent a two-bedroom apartment with a renewable yearly lease and a month-to-month lease thereafter. There was also an option to sign a two-year lease after six months of month-to-month leasing. No pets were allowed. The lease would start on March 15th to give them time to clean the apartment. Also, Michael would move in before the wedding.

Laura and Michael went back to Northend Hospital to pick up Laura's car.

"Laura, I'm going to follow you home."

"You don't have to, Michael. You look exhausted."

"I just want to be sure you get home safe."

"It is so nice to know that someone worries about my safety all the time."

"I know you worry about me, too."

"How do you know?"

"I can see it in your eyes."

"You do not only read minds, you also read body language! Let's go home now. Mom must be waiting for us. She is so excited about having you as a son-in-law."

"The feeling is mutual."

Laura drove ahead of Michael. The expressway was practically empty. It took them only thirty minutes to reach the Secula residence. Mrs. Secula was still awake. She was so happy to see Laura and Michael.

"You are such an attractive couple. You look so happy."

"Mom, we are indeed very happy and hope the happiness we feel now never wears off."

"I hope so, too. You deserve each other. Your father would have been very happy to have Michael for a son-in-law."

"I know he would. Michael reminds me of Dad in a lot of ways. Sometimes, it is so eerie; he even talks like Dad, too."

"I know."

"I hope I don't fail to meet your high expectations of me!"

"We have settled everything we need, Mom. All we have to do now is attend the Pre-Canaan Conference. I have to arrange my moonlighting schedule. I would like to work two nights a week at Southern Hospital until we are married. Once we are married, I would like to work there once a week. What do you think, Michael?"

"We have to discuss that later. I saw Dr. Jay Simmons in the hospital today. He told me that James Dillon would be flying back to Ireland three days after our wedding. He wants us to attend a sit-down dinner for James Dillon and his family. He thought it would be better for him to give the party ahead of time so that we could both attend."

"Dr. Simmons is a very thoughtful man."

"He is not just a thoughtful man. He cares deeply about all his residents and always goes out of his way to help them out, both professionally and personally. I would never hesitate to ask for his help if I had to."

"I am glad to hear that he is really good with the people he works with."

"We are so lucky to have met and known him."

"We have to see Father Walls tomorrow and finalize our Pre-Canaan Conference. We can probably call the rectory to save time."

"That would be fine with me."

Laura started yawning.

"Is that a signal that I should leave now?"

"You can stay as long as you want."

"Well, I better leave. I will talk to you tomorrow."

Laura walked Michael to the door and bade him good night.

She looked out the window and watched Michael drive away. She said to herself, "Thank you, God, for sending me Michael."

"Laura, are you talking to me?"

"No, Mom, I was just repeating something."

Laura went back to the kitchen; Mrs. Secula asked Laura to take a seat.

"We are going to have a heart-to-heart talk, mother to daughter. You have been so busy that I don't even get a chance to talk to you. Have you found an apartment yet?"

"Yes, we are going to live downtown in an apartment owned by the Jelton Corporation. It has two bedrooms. It will be big enough for us even if we have a child."

"Do you plan to have a baby while you are in training?"

"Mom, I am thirty, and Michael is thirty-three. We don't want to wait too long. Michael and I have discussed artificial contraception, but we don't believe in it. He himself can't understand why a man would subject his wife to future risk of stroke, hypertension, and breast cancer. He can't understand why a man would subject his wife to risks of Toxic Shock and death with the diaphragm and IUD. Michael is a very thoughtful and analytical man. We are going to look into Natural Family Planning; we hope to be able to plan our family."

"I am so happy for you. You are not marrying a macho man."

"I would not tolerate one, Mom. Mom, let us go to sleep. I have to wake up early tomorrow. Our operating room schedule is heavy. I probably will not even have a chance to talk to Michael until the afternoon. The only thing left for us to do is to attend the Pre-Canaan Conference. I will start working at Southern Hospital Monday."

CHAPTER XVIII

On January 15th, Laura rushed to Southern Hospital to work in the emergency room. Once she arrived there, there were about four patients left for her to examine.

In room one was an eight-year-old boy who had accidentally incurred lacerations on his chin when he had hit his face against a chair while playing.

In room six was a young 12-year-old boy with bee sting. He was given a steroid injection and antihistamine tablets to take home.

In room four was a 35-year-old man waiting to go to X-Ray with a possible fracture of the right leg.

In room eight was a 55-year-old cardiac patient waiting for a bed in the coronary care unit.

From room one, Laura could hear the ambulance siren. A young boy was being carried on a stretcher through the corridor by the rescue squad. The mother was hysterical. "Is my son still alive? Is he still breathing?"

Laura rushed to room three. She quickly examined the patient. She could not hear any heartbeat or feel the pulse. She took aside the distraught parents and sadly told them that their boy was dead.

"I am sorry, but there was nothing more we could do. Your son died of a condition called Epiglottitis (a life-threatening bacterial infection of the epiglottis causing airway obstruction). I wish he had been brought here sooner."

"We could not get through to the HMO doctor's office at nine o'clock. By ten o'clock, I was able to talk to the secretary and told her my son was having problems with sore throat and breathing. She told me to wait and bring the baby to the office at one-thirty."

"Did you talk to the doctor?"

"No, just to the secretary."

"Is that the procedure in this doctor's office?"

"Yes, I never talk to the doctor whenever I call. If I needed a referral to a specialist, I got a third degree from the secretary before I could get one. They make you feel like a second class citizen because you are HMO. It is really assembly line medicine. Sometimes, we waited two and a half to three hours for my children's check-ups."

"Well, I wish I could have helped your son. This is a coroner's case. I have to call the medical examiner's office and ask if your son should be autopsied here or in their office. Do you want something hot to drink?"

"Thank you, doctor. You have done more than enough for us. Thank you for your kindness."

"Please, stay here while I call all the authorities concerned. Don't try to control your feelings. Cry, if you want to cry. There is nothing more painful than losing a precious child. If you want to make phone calls, you can use the phone on the wall. Just dial nine. I will be back shortly. If you need something, just let me know."

Laura called the coroner's office. "I have a three year-old boy who has been brought in DOA. The mother has given me a sketchy summary. She is all shaken up. The father could not even talk about this misfortune."

The man at the coroner's office said, "We will pick up the body in an hour. Be sure all the necessary papers are signed."

"Thank you, sir."

Laura went back to the couple. "I have straightened out everything. Here's the phone number of the coroner's office. You can call them anytime if you have questions. You can also call me at my regular work place if you have any questions."

"Thank you, Dr. Secula."

Laura took their address and phone number. "Please, don't hesitate to call me any time if I can be of help."

Laura gripped their hands tightly and said goodbye. "Take care." Then she said to herself, "This HMO insurance stinks. HMO does not cut healthcare cost; it does, though, cut lives."

Laura was examining the patient with a fractured right arm in room five, when the rescue squad brought in a gunshot wound victim. The patient was an eight-month pregnant cop whose husband had shot her during an altercation. Laura quickly got the fetal doppler to listen to the baby. The fetal heartbeat was strong and regular. The patient's vital signs were stable. An intravenous line was immediately started.

The obstetrician on call was notified immediately. Blood studies were immediately drawn, and the patient was rushed to the delivery room. The patient was readied for an emergency Caesarean section.

An hour later, Laura called the delivery room.

"How is the patient with the gunshot wound doing?"

"The bullet went straight through the fundus of the uterus into the placenta. The part of the placenta in which the bullet lodged had a big clot due to the shearing of the placenta. The baby and the mother are both fine."

"Is she going to press charges against her husband?"

"I don't think so. The husband is here now with her parents."

"I see," Laura paused and thanked the head nurse.

As soon as Laura put down the phone, an ambulance whisked in a 16-year-old girl with vaginal bleeding. This patient was nine months pregnant. She had just shot up her left arm with coke at a party. She started having abdominal cramps and vaginal bleeding immediately after injecting herself. Her boyfriend, who was also under the influence of illicit drugs, called the ambulance.

Laura had a hard time obtaining the medical history from the patient and from her boyfriend. She immediately started her on an intravenous line with a large bore needle. She ordered the nurse to take the patient to the delivery room immediately. Laura extracted the blood herself and asked one of the nurse's aides to take the blood to the laboratory immediately.

Dr. Sawyer, the obstetrician who had sectioned the patient with the gunshot wound, was waiting in the delivery room, ready to examine and proceed with emergency management of the young primigravida with abruptio placenta secondary to illicit drugs. This patient had been previously registered in another clinic. The head nurse called the delivery room of that clinic and was able to obtain some information about her prenatal care.

Dr. Sawyer did an emergency Caesarean section. In surgery, the placenta was about two thirds detached from the wall of the uterus; the baby's apgar was six. The neonatologist resuscitated the baby. The baby had the typical shrill cry of an infant with Withdrawal Syndrome. The baby was rushed immediately to the neonatal intensive care unit.

"Please call the laboratory. I want all the blood studies repeated. I want a urine sample tested for recreational drugs, too. It is a shame that some young people get involved with drugs. This poor baby has already partially lost a battle for survival! What can you do? Do you turn in these pregnant women to the cops or do you rehabilitate them? Drug abuse among pregnant women is one of the main causes of infant morbidity and mortality. There is no way we can improve our infant mortality rate, unless we deal with our social issues."

"I don't know what the answer is, Dr. Sawyer. I think we should start with our fragmented family unit first and go from there," said the head nurse.

"I do, too. Kids have no role models anymore."

"I could not agree more."

The emergency room was now packed to capacity. Five burn victims were brought into the accident ward. Three children, whose bodies had been burned sixty percent, were transferred to the hospital burn center after they had been stabilized. The two other burn victims were sent home after treatment.

It was almost time for Laura to take off, but her relief did not make it; his wife had gone into premature labor. Laura had to stay another eight hours.

Michael called Laura.

"Michael, I can't talk now. I am swamped with patients."

"I just wanted to tell you that Dr. Simmons invited us to dinner next Friday. A visiting medical professor will be coming to his house, and he wants this doctor to meet some of his residents. I'll tell you all about it tomorrow. Bye."

"Please, don't call me tomorrow. I will call you. Bye."

As soon as Laura hung up, the nurse called her.

"Dr. Secula, there is an elderly lady who has to be seen immediately in room four."

Laura rushed to room four. "My God, how could anyone do this to this sweet old lady? Please call the surgeon immediately. This lady needs emergency surgery. Please tell him this lady has prolapsed colon through a ruptured vagina. Please get me some towels and moisten them with warm saline. I will have to cover this bowel with them."

Laura started an intravenous line and prophylactic antibiotics. She immediately talked to the family about the patient's medical condition.

The daughter was hysterical. "Who could have done this to my mother? She doesn't deserve this."

"Did you report this incident to the cops?"

"Yes, but I had to leave with the ambulance. Our neighbor gave all the information to the police. There were some jewelry and money missing. What is really strange is that the red robe she was wearing is missing as well."

"I have also called a gynecologist to check your mother and take some specimen to see if your mother was molested."

"I can't believe this. I can't believe that there is a human being who could inflict such harm on a sweet elderly lady. I just can't."

"I understand what you are trying to say, but some people are irrational because they are under the influence of drugs. They can't control themselves."

"You mean to say, this is drug related?"

"Most probably. Your mother told me that the burglar was a young man, obviously on drugs, who used to mow your lawn."

"My God, I know this kid! I know his family! His family is nice; I could never imagine that this kid would do this to my mother."

"This kid might be basically a nice kid. He probably got into drugs because of peer pressure. Drug addiction does not discriminate. It is a myth that only poor people get involved with drugs. Doctors, lawyers, nurses, and people from every stratum of society get involved with drugs. Our country is under siege from drugs. The best way to fight the drug war is by cutting the demand! There is no way we can win the war on drugs unless we start solving social problems. People take illegal drugs when they are unhappy, bored, sad, or when misfortune befalls them. On the other hand, people sell drugs because it is the easiest way to make money. It is a vicious cycle. I don't know what the solution will be."

"I don't know either."

Both the surgeon and gynecologist on call came at the same time. They both decided that the patient should be taken down to the operating room immediately. The gynecologist decided that he should do the pelvic examination in the operating room while he prepped the perineum for surgery. Both the surgeon and the gynecologist explained to the daughter the anticipated surgical procedure and the risks involved with the surgery and anaesthesia.

"We will get in touch with you as soon as we are done. You can either wait around the emergency room or in the lobby."

"Thank you, doctors."

Mrs. Ann Murray was very cooperative. She was in good shape healthwise, in spite of the fact that she was 71-years-old.

Dr. Sawyer inserted a sterile vaginal pack and decided to do the vaginal repair intra-abdominally. He was going to assist Dr. Bismarck with the exploratory laparotomy. During the exploration, it was noted that a part of the bowel was ruptured. Vaginal repair and control of the bleeding were done, as well as a colostomy. The operation was finished without any incident.

Dr. Sawyer and Dr. Bismarck talked to Mrs. Murray's daughter after the surgery.

"We could not do much for your Mom today. We repaired the vaginal rupture and did a colostomy. A bowel resection will be done later. Your Mom will be moving her bowels through her colostomy. A stoma nurse will teach you on how to take care of the colostomy. If you have any questions, please don't hesitate to call me. I do not know yet how long your mother will be in the hospital."

"Thank you, doctors. Thank you for your immediate response when Dr. Secula called you. It is really a big load off my shoulders knowing that my mother is in stable condition. Good morning to you both."

A nurse ran up to Laura and said, "Dr. Secula, Dr. Secula, please come to room three. Please hurry!"

Laura rushed to room three. "What's the matter?"

"This patient's blood pressure is 200/120. Her skin is getting hard and leathery. Her whole back is leathery, but not tender. In her history, she stated that she used a dry-shampoo spray."

"Please get me 240 mg of Solu-Medrol and Nipride STAT. We have to send this patient to the ICU. Did you get any blood test result yet?"

"Yes, the Eosinophile count is markedly elevated."

What we have here is an Acute Disseminated Necrotizing Fasciitis. She has had an allergic reaction to yellow fragrance # 5. You have to put in a STAT call to an internist. She should be seen immediately and monitored closely in ICU."

"I have already put in a call to the internist. His answering service took the message."

"Please call back the answering service. Tell the operator it's an emergency and that the doctor should get in touch with me here."

"I will do that, Dr. Secula."

A little later, Dr. Reeves walked in. "Dr. Secula, I heard you were looking for me."

"Yes, Dr. Reeves. We have a very sick patient with Acute Disseminated Necrotizing Fasciitis. I gave her Solu-Medrol and Lasix I.V. and started her on Nipride to treat her Acute Malignant Hypertension."

"How sure are you of your diagnosis?"

"I am positive. The clincher is the leathery skin and markedly elevated Eosinophile count. I have read some case reports in the medical and surgical journals, too."

"I am impressed. I have never seen a case like this. Do you remember in what journal you read about these cases?"

"I read a lot of journals to keep up with the advances in medicine. The best book to find out about literature research is the *Index Medicus*. Just look under 'Necrotizing Fasciitis.' There is another type wherein the patient develops a fulminant infection after an invasive procedure. It could prove fatal if the doctor does not recognize it early enough to aggressively treat the patient. It can also be a preventable catastrophe; the mortality rate in diabetics is high, though, 50-80 percent. It can occur in post-irradiated patients, too. It is scary to even think about this disease in postpartum patients because pregnant women are immunosuppressed."

"What is the best way to handle it in pregnant women and patients undergoing surgery or invasive procedures?"

"Do more cultures pre-operatively and post-operatively. If a physician does it pre-operatively, he or she will be able to differentiate between commensal, iatrogenic, or nosocomial infections. It is not only good medicine, it protects the patient's life and the doctor's, too."

"Do you think we can do that with cost-containment by the government and the insurance companies?"

"We should not let cost-containment influence our medical judgement. Our primary goal should be good patient care."

"I agree with you totally. It is time for organized medicine to stand up for its patients."

"I am glad you understand my point. All the HMO plans are anti-Hippocratic. Any physician who gets sued for following the HMO guidelines will be in an untenable position. All the plaintiff lawyer has to point out to the jury is that the patient suffered or died because of the inhumane treatment rendered to him or her due to the financial incentives involved."

"I am glad I am not an HMO participant."

"Good for you."

"Dr. Secula, it has been a pleasure talking to you and thank you, too, for the pearls! I will never forget a case like this. I will also check the *Index Medicus* and the literature on Necrotizing Fasciitis."

"Thank you."

Laura was quite exhausted. Finally, all the patients were discharged. The rest of the patients seen were waiting for admission.

It did not take Laura that long to reach Northend Hospital. She passed through the emergency room. The trauma unit was jammed. There had been a shooting spree in a nearby restaurant. There were three casualties. Two wounded patients were being readied for the operating room. The chief resident saw Laura.

"Laura, we need an extra hand in the operating room."

"I will be there. I am just going to change and get a cup of coffee."

"I know I can depend on you. We should be in the operating room in fifteen minutes."

"See you then."

The patient, a fortyish, heavyset woman, was just being wheeled to the operating room when Laura came down.

"Laura, could you shave the abdomen while I get scrubbed? There are not enough nurses to help us out. Another room has to be opened for the other patient. He is almost bled out.

The first year resident is pumping four units of blood now. I called the attending physician to come in and scrub with the first year resident."

"No problem, I will shave and prep the whole abdomen, too."

"Thanks."

Laura and Dr. Saltine explored the patient's abdomen. Three thousand cc of blood were suctioned. The bleeding was coming from the liver. The liver was gently sutured. Bleeding from the liver persisted. Thrombin was sprayed on the liver area; however, the bleeding persisted. Avitene was placed on the site of the bleeding, but still the bleeding persisted.

"My God, we are going to lose this patient. I think this patient has a diseased liver or missing blood factor. We might be dealing with Von Willebrand disease." (a congenital disorder due to deficient platelet function and factor VIII).

"Please call the hematologist. Get the laboratory and tell them to give us two units of fresh frozen plasma. Draw the blood for hemorrhagic studies, bleeding time, platelet count, and factor VIII. Tell the laboratory that we will need cryoprecipitate, too."

The hematologist arrived in fifteen minutes. He ran the tests immediately. The patient's fibrinogen was zero. The platelet count was 75,000 per cubic mm.; the norm was 110,000-400,000 per cubic mm. The hematologist sent up two units of fresh frozen plasma and six units of cryoprecipitate.

All of a sudden, the bleeding from the liver slowed down to an ooze.

"Let's spray the thrombin solution again."

"Please get us a vial of thrombin powder and dilute it," Laura said to the scrub nurse.

Laura sprayed the thrombin solution on the oozing site.

"It is slowing down now. Let's wait. The laboratory just sent up six units more of cryoprecipitate. Let's hope this oozing will completely stop."

"We have to inspect the other organs to see if there is any damage. The spleen, kidneys, and stomach are all fine. We have to run the whole length of both the small and large intestines."

"Let's close while we are ahead. Let's have one last look at the liver."

"The liver area is dry. Let's get the sponge count."

"First sponge count is correct."

"Four kellys, please, and Dexon sutures."

"Second sponge, instrument, and needle count are all correct."

"Dressings, please. Thanks to everyone."

Laura and Dr. Saltine went to the waiting room to talk to the husband of the patient.

"Everything went well. Your wife will be transferred to the ICU after she is reacted. She has to be monitored closely. She lost a lot of blood. We had to give her a blood factor transfusion. We had no choice. The blood factor transfusion helped us stop the bleeding. She had us scared for a while, but, eventually, the bleeding from the sutured laceration was completely stopped."

"Thank you, doctors."

"You are welcome."

Laura and Dr. Saltine went to the next room where the other victim was being operated on. The bullet had lodged into the patient's heart. The cardiovascular surgeon had to be called in to suture the heart. The patient's pericardium was filled with blood. This was suctioned. The patient did well during the surgery and was moved to the coronary intensive care unit. He would be followed by the cardiovascular surgeon and cardiologist.

"Are we going to have Journal Club this afternoon?"

"I will have to cancel it. Everyone is exhausted and sleepy. I will reschedule it for next week."

"I have to go to the surgical clinic. I have about fifty patients to see. I hope the second year residents will be able to help me."

"I will tell them to go to the surgical clinic as soon as they get finished in the operating room."

"Thank you."

It was already two o'clock, and the second year residents had not arrived at the clinic yet. Laura had already seen fifteen post-operative check-ups. The rest were all new patients who were still filling out the history questionnaires. By two-fifteen, the other residents had arrived.

"Guys, I will give each of you sixteen patients to see. I have already seen eighteen patients. We will be seeing a total of fifty patients today. I have to go to the ward as soon as I see all my patients. I have to make rounds."

"Thank you for covering for us, Laura. We owe you one."

"You are welcome."

Laura went to the ward to make rounds. All her patients were doing well. The elderly man whose gallbladder she had operated on was doing better with his diabetes. He should be ready to go home in two to three days as soon as his blood sugar was stabilized. She then went to see Mrs. Springfield in the next room.

"How are you, Mrs. Springfield? I have good news for you. All the fifteen lymph nodes taken from your axilla are negative. I am very happy and optimistic for you."

"Thank you, Dr. Secula."

"I will have to refer you to a medical oncologist. He will decide whether you will need further therapy as soon as we get the estrogen receptor assay. In the meantime, I want you to read all this layman literature about breast cancer. I would like to talk to your husband, too, to see if he has any questions or fears about your condition. Sometimes, men have a hard time accepting breast cancer. The three of us can discuss all your questions; write them down so you won't forget."

"Thank you, Dr. Secula."

"I am going to my call room to get some sleep. Before visiting hours are over, please have the nurse ring my room. I would be more than happy to talk to your husband about your illness."

Laura woke up at eight-thirty in the evening. She was not sure whether her phone rang or not. She decided to go back to Mrs. Springfield's room.

"Dr. Secula, I decided not to have the nurse call you. My husband was very distraught. He cried so hard! I did not know whether they were tears of joy or sadness. I do not know whether he is grieving the loss of my breast or whether he is happy to know that my chances of survival are better because the type of cancer I have doesn't involve my lymph glands."

"It is probably both. I'm sure he feels very badly for you, too, because of the pain you are having right now."

"I know. We have been married for twenty-five years, and this is the first time I have been hospitalized except for three childbirths."

"Do you have any daughters?"

"No, I have three sons. They are all happily married right now. I have two sisters, though."

"Please tell your sisters to get mammography requests from their physicians."

"I have already told them. I wish I had had my mammography done sooner. I was trying to save money for it. My healthcare insurance did not pay for it two and a half years ago. So I waited, and this is the result of my waiting too long, especially since cancer cells are usually present in the breast several years before a mass will show in a mammogram."

"I am sorry to hear that. Every spring some hospitals in the Philadelphia area offer mammogram screening which is subsidized by the American Cancer Society."

"I have heard about this cancer screening. I called three hospitals but none of them could take me because their quotas were filled up."

"I will be getting the final report of the permanent tissue section tomorrow. I will be back to explain to you what the pathology report means."

"Thank you, Dr. Secula."

Laura called Michael. "I am sorry, but I just woke up a while ago and I had to go back to the surgical ward to talk to Mrs. Springfield. Mr. Springfield was so upset that he had to leave before he could talk to me. I took his number. I am going to call him at home as soon as I hang up."

"I would be very upset, too, if my wife developed breast cancer."

"I know you would. I better call Mr. Springfield before he goes to sleep."

"I will see you Friday. I will pick you up at seven o'clock."

"Do we have to bring anything?"

"Yes, but I will take care of that."

"Thank you, Michael."

After hanging up, Laura dialed Mr. Springfield.

"Mr. Springfield, I am sorry to bother you this late. I am Laura Secula. I'm taking care of your wife."

"I know all about you. My wife speaks very highly of you."

"I assume that Mrs. Springfield has told you about the diagnosis."

"Yes, she did."

"Mr. Springfield, I just want to let you know how sorry I am about your wife's situation. I fault the healthcare insurance company for refusing to pay for a mammography. It is terrible! Healthcare insurance companies care only about the bottom line. Your wife's cancer could have been detected earlier, if she had been X-Rayed sooner. This is an unfortunate incident. She needs a lot of moral support and encouragement. I know you will understand. There are times that she will feel irritable, depressed, and sorry for herself. You have to put up with all her moods. You can really help her by being supportive and by showing her that you are strong. Just show her you care and love her. Be positive."

"I intend to do that, Dr. Secula."

"I know I can count on you. If you have any questions, please don't hesitate to call me."

"I will do that, Dr. Secula. Thank you for calling me and thank you for your time."

Laura went back to sleep.

CHAPTER XIX

Michael was at the Secula residence at exactly seven o'clock. Laura was dressed in a beautiful blue chiffon dress with a pearl necklace. Michael, as usual, was in a blue wool suit. They made a stunning couple.

Both kissed Mrs. Secula good night before they left. Jeanie was out with her friends.

"Be careful driving and have a nice time. I hope it does not snow on your way back home."

"We hope so, too."

Michael and Laura had a leisurely drive through the countryside before reaching Dr. Simmons' home. Everyone was enjoying the cocktail hour by the time they arrived. Dr. Simmons introduced Michael and Laura to the distinguished professor from Oxford University, Dr. Delfinder. Mrs. Delfinder was quite charming and had an aristocratic look, very dignified and elegant.

Estela and Jorge, James Dillon, John Miller, and their wives were also there in addition to the other professors from the university. Debbie Simmons was mingling with the other guests.

Estela and Jorge were doing well in Miami, Florida. Most of their patients were compatriots. They were going to stay at the Simmons home for the weekend and then proceed to New York to look for a modeling school for Estela's cousin, Ditas.

The group decided to sit together for dinner. It was just like a reunion. They also had sat together at Dr. Simmons' retirement party.

"James, when are you going back to Ireland?"

"We are just waiting to attend Michael and Laura's wedding. We are going to leave March 21st. We are going to stop over in England and Scotland for two weeks. We might not be able to travel as often as we would like because I will be teaching at Trinity University and Michelle will be home full time to take care of the baby."

John Miller added, "I am going to practice in Ohio. I am going to join another doctor who finished his residency in the university and was also trained by Dr. Simmons."

"Come and visit us in Florida whenever you have a chance. Debbie is going there on her vacation before she starts working at the medical examiner's office."

"Michael, where are you going for your honeymoon?"

"We are going to Hawaii for a week. Then we will go back to work after we fix our apartment."

"Are you planning to go into private practice after you finish your fellowship?"

"I don't know yet. Laura has one and a half years more to go. We have to wait and see. Father John would love to see me and Laura practice in Indiana, but I don't think Laura is keen on that."

Laura just smiled and did not say a word.

"These tables are so exquisitely set. I bet Debbie did all the flower arrangements, too. She has such impeccable taste."

"That's an understatement."

Dr. Simmons came over to their table.

"Dr. Delfinder and I will be waiting for all of you in the library. You can ask any questions you want. He is an Emeritus Professor in surgery at Oxford University. He is also well-versed on healthcare issues. I can more or less guess he will be asked a lot of questions about the National Health Insurance in England."

"You are right on target, Dr. Simmons!" everyone said in unison.

As soon as everyone was done with dessert, they all proceeded to the study room. Dr. Delfinder sat at the center of the study table. The rest of the twenty doctors and their wives seated themselves on the other side of the table.

"I understand you are all interested in finding out about our healthcare system."

"Yes, we are."

"Well, our healthcare system is not running as well as the news and television media have portrayed. We have the same shortage of nurses as you do. We don't have enough cytotechnicians to screen pap smears. It takes about six months to get a pap smear report back. We have antiquated medical equipment. We don't have as much sophisticated technology as you, like Ultrasounds, CAT Scans, and MRI's. It takes longer for testing to be done in England than in the U.S. The medicolegal system is different and better. Depositions and pretrial hearings are only allowed on special decrees. There is a special committee that screens medical malpractice suits. Only meritorious cases go on trial. No frivolous suits are filed. This has cut the cost of defensive medicine which, I think, runs to about $45 billion in your country."

"You are absolutely right," said Dr. Simmons.

John Miller asked, "Is it fair to compare healthcare cost in England and the U.S. then?"

"No, because our medico-legal system is different from yours. In spite of the good points of our healthcare system, though, it is still not working. It is about to collapse. We have a big federal deficit like you. The government is about to adopt the worst part of your healthcare system, the HMO's! God help the British people!"

Michael exclaimed, "Isn't it ironic that both governments want to adopt each other's bad healthcare system?"

"Don't worry about it. Private practice in England has survived; private practice in the United States will survive, too."

"We hope so."

It was Dr. Simmons' turn to speak, "The media have duped the public into believing that either the Canadian or British healthcare system will be good for the American people. A National Healthcare Plan is not feasible in the United States. First of all, Americans are basically impatient; they would not be willing to wait the six months that Canadians do for the results of a CAT Scan or pap smear. Secondly, to have a National Healthcare Plan, income tax would have to increase by 14%, payroll tax by 15-29%, and consumption tax by 9-10%. Americans wouldn't like that either."

It was Laura's turn to speak, "The media are trying to compare apples and oranges. Canada has only about 25 million people compared to the United States' 250 million. We have more elderly people here. There are no slums in Canada. Our healthcare system is under siege by our social problems, like drugs, AIDS, poverty, sexually transmitted diseases, and poor nutrition. Also, our flawed healthcare policies are costing more money for administrative cost. Thirty percent of each healthcare dollar is spent on paper work. Every doctor and hospital is trying to survive. Charity, compassion, and altruism have been replaced by the bottom line and greed. It is very hard for an uninsured patient to find a doctor who will operate on her or him for free. Greed and fraud are rampant in the healthcare industry. There are too many business ventures being pushed by doctors themselves, like medical equipment and unnecessary testing in their offices in order to increase the doctor's shrinking revenue. Organized medicine has failed the public! I see it every day. Some doctors feel they are not accountable to the public. We really have to rebuild our image."

"What is your opinion, Dr. Dillon?"

"I could not agree more with what Laura has said. Our reputation is really under fire. This will really be well-publicized when financial incentives for HMO go on trial in Philadelphia.

I am sure this trial will be followed by the national media and Physicians Who Care. This is an organization of 3,000 doctors who believe in freedom of choice, and affordable and accessible healthcare for everyone. It believes in quality care and that the patient should be the first priority, not the doctor's pocketbook. It is trying to launch a grassroots campaign to educate the public about the healthcare crisis."

"What a lofty goal!"

"More power to these doctors if they can do it. It is very hard to educate an indifferent public."

"I know."

It was almost eleven o'clock. Dr. Delfinder was looking at his watch, "I guess it is time for us to leave. We have to be at the airport at seven in the morning. This has been a wonderful evening for me, meeting and talking to all of you young, idealistic doctors. I hope you do not change."

"May I offer you a ride, Dr. Delfinder?"

"Thank you, Dr. Olsire, but the hotel is going to send the limousine to pick us up."

"Would you like to have some coffee while you are waiting for your limousine?"

"No, thank you. I am going to leave my address with Dr. Simmons. If any of you happens to be traveling in England, please look me up. I will be pleased to give you a tour of the university and show you around town. Good night, everyone."

All the guests left except Estela and Jorge.

CHAPTER XX

Laura made rounds early Saturday. She went to the pathology laboratory to check on the slides of Mrs. Springfield. The permanent sections of her breast tissues were done. There were no metastases in any of the lymph nodes sampled. She requested an oncologist to see if Mrs. Springfield would need chemotherapy or Tamoxifen pending the hormonal receptor test result.

Laura went to see Mrs. Springfield in her room.

"I have good news for you, Mrs. Springfield. The permanent breast tissue sections showed no metastases in the sampled lymph nodes. The medical oncologist will see you and make a decision whether you need chemotherapy or Tamoxifen depending on the result of the estrogen and progesterone receptors. He will explain to you why you need it and the risks involved in taking either the Tamoxifen or chemotheraphy."

"Thank you, Dr. Secula."

"Have a nice weekend, Mrs. Springfield. I will be back tomorrow to make rounds."

Laura rushed home. She, her mom, and Jeanie were going for their final trousseau fittings. She had another night to work in the accident ward before the wedding. She was starting to get jittery. She planned to go shopping with Michael tomorrow to buy some stuff for Father John.

The bridal shop was crowded when they arrived. They had to wait an hour before they could try their gowns. All their gowns fitted very easily. The only problem was that Laura's headdress needed retouching. Otherwise, everything went well. Laura dropped by the mall on their way home to buy some calligraphy ink. She and Jeanie wanted to write out the seating arrangement cards in calligraphy.

Michael arrived at the Secula residence by nine in the morning the next day.

"Michael, did you have breakfast?"

"I did, but I would appreciate a cup of coffee with sugar and milk."

"It is coming."

"Thank you. Are your mom and Jeanie awake yet?"

"No, we slept late. We did the seating arrangement cards. Everything is done. I just have to buy presents for the bridal party. The flowers have all been ordered, too."

"Thank God, I don't have to worry about anything. How lucky can I be!"

"You bet you are. You are about to win a big jackpot, and that's me!"

"I know it!"

Laura and Michael went to the mall on Roosevelt Boulevard.

"Laura, I think the lady inside that store is Patty Singleton."

"I don't think so. She just looks like Patty. Her hair is different and she is too skinny."

"Let's go inside and say hello."

Laura and Michael approached Patty.

"Patty, how are you?"

"I'm Mrs. Singleton to you. Euridis, let's go. I don't have to talk to these two strangers."

Laura and Michael were both dumbfounded.

"My God, what's going on with Patty? I must call Mrs. Collins to find out what's wrong with Patty. She's had a sudden change of personality and is hostile, too."

"Don't worry, Michael. She probably is still very depressed and is trying to blot out the memory of Charlie's death. And, everytime she sees you, you remind her of Charlie and his protracted, agonizing illness."

"I hope she does not have anything as serious as a brain tumor that's causing a change in her personality."

"I hope so, too."

"Let's get going so that I can call Mrs. Collins as soon as we get home. We only have to buy some bed sheets, towels, and pillows."

"We have to go to the houseware outlet store then."

"No problem."

On their way home, Michael could not stop talking about Patty.

"You know, Charlie gave me three letters before he died, two for me and one for Patty. I wonder what was in the letter that Charlie asked me to give to Patty after his death."

"I don't know."

"This is strange, too. I am not supposed to open my letters for two years."

"Where did you put them?"

"I don't know. We would not be able to open them now, anyway. We have to follow the wish of a dead person."

"This is an enigma!"

"I know. I can't understand why Charlie left me those letters."

"When you get home, please look for them. Your life or career might be at stake."

"I understand your concern."

As soon as they arrived at the Secula residence, Michael tried to call Mrs. Collins, but the phone was disconnected.

"What are we going to do now?"

"I have to drop by their house and find out what is going on."

"Do you want me to come with you?"

"No, just stay home and rest."

Michael drove down to Vestar Street, and parked in front of Mrs. Collins' house. The house had a SOLD sign in front of it.

Michael went around the neighborhood and tried to ask where Patty and her mom had moved. Nobody could tell him where they had moved. He took down the realtor's phone number. Early Monday morning, Michael called the realtor to find out if he knew the new address of Patty and Mrs. Collins.

The realtor told Michael that Patty had moved to an apartment. Mrs. Collins had gone to a nursing home because she could not move the wheelchair anymore. She was totally incapacitated with her arthritis.

"How about Patty's daughters?"

"I don't know where they are."

"Does Patty drive a car?"

"I don't think so."

"How about the girls?"

"Michelle has a second-hand car which she drives around. She and Kathy are both in college."

"Do you know what college they attend?"

"No, I wish I did."

"I am going to leave you my phone number in case you see either Kathy or Michelle. Please, tell them I have been looking for them. Please give them my number."

"I will do that."

"Thanks a lot."

"You are welcome."

As soon as Michael reached his apartment, he called Laura.

"It's bad news. Nobody knows where Patty lives. Mrs. Collins lives in a nursing home now. The girls are both in college. Nobody, though, knows their addresses. It is kind of strange."

"Don't worry, Michael. Sooner or later, we will find them."

"I hope so. I worry about Mrs. Collins. She must be very lonely in the nursing home. I wish I knew where she was. We would at least be able to visit her."

"I know how you feel, Michael. Probably we could call all the nursing homes in Philadelphia. I will call half of them, all the ones located in the Northeast. Sears and Roebuck should be our dividing line."

"That's fine with me."

An hour later, Michael called Laura.

"I found out where Mrs. Collins is."

"Where?"

"At the Bellwood Nursing Home, but she is in bad shape. She can't talk anymore. She had a stroke two weeks ago."

"Let's go and see her tomorrow then. I will pick you up at home at seven o'clock in the evening."

"That will be fine."

The next day, Michael was late in picking up Laura. So, by the time Laura and Michael reached the nursing home, visiting hours were almost over.

Michael spotted Patty in the parking lot with Euridis. He tried to wave at her. Patty completely ignored him and drove away with Euridis.

"Michael, don't get upset about Patty. We will find out later why she is acting weird."

Michael talked the nurse supervisor into letting them in.

"Are you Dr. Olsire?"

"Yes, I am. Why?"

"Mrs. Collins wrote this letter for you two weeks ago before she had the stroke."

"Michael, let's read it."

Dear Dr. Olsire,

I can't thank you enough for all your kindnesses and thoughtfulness to us. Patty told me that, when she saw you in the mall a few weeks ago, she did not talk to you because you did not notice her. I wish to apologize for Patty's rude behavior towards you. I can't understand why she's changed suddenly. She works with this woman Euridis at the law firm of a Robert Smith. Please, forgive my daughter for all her rudeness towards you. She is not herself.

Sincerely,
Ann Collins

Michael almost choked after he read the letter.

"How can Patty do this to Charlie? He might be the same Robert Smith who caused Charlie's AIDS and the AIDS of the five homeless people who are now confined in the university hospital. Sometimes people really do weird things. I can't figure this one out."

"I can't either. Probably this is not the same Robert Smith that Charlie used to talk about."

"I can't think anymore. I am so confused."

"Let's see Mrs. Collins."

Mrs. Collins was unresponsive when Michael touched and squeezed her right hand, but she tried to signal to Michael and Laura to sit.

Michael and Laura both nodded. Mrs. Collins tried to reach for a glass of water. Michael sat her up and helped her drink through the straw. She smiled at Michael and tried to squeeze his hand, but she could not do it. Tears rolled down her cheeks. Laura took a tissue from her pocketbook and wiped Mrs. Collins' tears. Laura tried to comb Mrs. Collins' hair. She wiped her face with a wet wash cloth. Mrs. Collins smiled approvingly. She squeezed Laura's left hand. Laura tried to hold back her tears. She looked at Michael with a pained expression. She could see that Michael was misty-eyed, too. Mrs. Collins started crying.

"Mrs. Collins, don't worry. Laura and I will visit you again. We will be getting married in one week. We will visit you again as soon as we get back from Hawaii."

Mrs. Collins looked at both of them and smiled.

It was now nine o'clock. The supervisor approached them and told them that it was time for them to leave. Laura and Michael both kissed Mrs. Collins good night.

Mrs. Collins looked at them while they walked away.

"Laura, this is a terrible place to be at the twilight of one's life. People who stay here must be so lonely."

"I am sure some of them are here because everyone in the family has to go to work or because they have no family or because they are the only survivors."

"I wish the state and federal government would have a surprise inspection of nursing homes. Some of the homes are so filthy. Some of them are not even safe to live in. Some of them are so short of help that some patients fall off their beds and injure themselves. Some of them overmedicate patients so that patients will be asleep all the time."

"The family pays top dollar, you know, and the money has to be put up front."

"We must find a better way of taking care of our elderly."

"I know. I think we are the biggest cause of what's wrong in our healthcare system. As you have said before, there is so much greed in the healthcare industry."

"A nurse I met at the university hospital used to work in a nursing home owned by a physician. She quit her job because she could not stand working in such a dirty, maggot- and roach-infested nursing home."

"Really?"

"Yes, and the doctor would not even hire an exterminator to kill the bugs."

"How atrocious!"

"Also, the nurse I met had to help clean the kitchen when it got flooded because of a broken pipe, and she was scared to death of the maggots and roaches floating in the water."

"You are putting me on!"

"No, this is what this nurse told me. She is now working as a utilization reviewer for an insurance company. I don't think she'll ever work again in a nursing home after her bad experience."

CHAPTER XXI

On Sunday afternoon, Laura and Michael went to the airport to pick up Father John. His flight was delayed for twenty minutes.

"I'm quite worried. There is heavy snow in Indiana. I hope nothing is wrong with the plane."

"I hope so, too. The airline company would have made an announcement if something had been wrong with the plane. It must only be a delayed take off. Be optimistic, Michael."

"Let's get something to drink."

Laura and Michael went to the snack shop.

"Michael, look at the headline."

The headline read: "Robert Smith, the eminent medical malpractice lawyer, a possible candidate for municipal judge!"

"My God, if this man is Charlie's Robert Smith, he should be stopped!"

"How can we stop him? We are the only people who know that he might be the same person who is a drug-trafficker that has wrought havoc on homeless people."

"We can find out."

"How?"

"We will attend his fund-raising campaign in case he decides to run."

"That's a good idea."

"Flight 003 from Indianapolis, Indiana, is about to land," a voice on the loudspeaker announced.

"Michael, Father John is here."

"Let's go to gate three."

Father John waved at Michael and Laura.

"Michael, I'm over here!"

Michael and Laura walked towards Father John. Father John kissed Laura and Michael.

"It's so nice to finally meet you, Laura. You two really make a handsome couple."

"Father John, I would like you to meet my family. We will take you home to have dinner with us."

"I will be delighted."

The drive to the Secula residence from the airport did not take that long. The Schuylkill Expressway was practically empty. In thirty minutes, they were at the Secula residence.

Mrs. Secula and Jeanie were preparing dinner.

"Mom and Jeanie, I want you to meet Father John."

"Good evening, Father. We have heard a lot about you from Michael. He told us how much you've sacrificed in order to raise him to become such a nice man."

"I just did what I had to do."

"We are so grateful for Michael, Father."

"Father, do you want anything to drink?"

"No, thank you. I do not want to spoil my appetite."

"Dinner will be ready soon."

"Do you want white or red wine with your dinner?"

"White wine will be fine."

"Father, please sit at the head of the table. Michael will be sitting next to Laura."

"Let us say grace. God, bless this food of which we are about to partake. This is such a delicious looking meal! I have not had a good Italian meal since my elderly cook passed away."

"Who is cooking at the convent now, Father?"

"No one in particular. Some church volunteers rotate every third week. The parish can't afford to foot any extra bill. Our church collection has markedly gone down. Most of the younger population has moved away."

"This is true everywhere in the country. There are even Catholic parochial schools being closed. There is no such thing anymore as exclusive girls' or boys' parochial schools."

"That's a shame."

"Getting away from the subject for a moment, Father, are we going to have the dress rehearsal on Thursday?"

"Yes, Michael. I think that would be fine."

"I think it would be better if Michael canceled the post-rehearsal dinner reservation at the restaurant. Don't you, Mom? We will just have dinner here!"

"That's a good idea, Laura. Jeanie and I can manage to cook for twenty people."

"That would be too much work for you."

"Not at all."

"I will have to call everyone tonight," said Laura.

"You don't have to call Estela and Jorge. They are still in New York."

"When will they be back?"

"I think they are going to Dr. Simmons' house directly from New York. They will go back to Florida after the wedding."

"That will be one less call to make."

"Dessert will be ready soon."

"Who wants coffee or tea?"

"I will have tea, Mrs. Secula."

"Father, would you prefer chocolate cake or Italian Rum Cake?"

"I will take a small slice of each."

After the meal, Father John said, "Thank you for such a delicious dinner."

"Mrs. Secula, I think we better get going. Father needs to rest."

"He must be tired from his flight," said Laura.

"Mrs. Secula, Laura, and Jeanie, thank you very much. I will be seeing you soon."

"Good night, Father. Good night, Michael."

"Good night."

Michael and Father John drove leisurely to University City.

"Michael, I am very impressed with Laura. She is a strong-willed lady, and she has a mind of her own."

"Father John, Laura has character. She is unique, and she has great self-esteem."

"I can tell by the way she talks, and it shows with her body language, too. You are both very lucky to have met each other."

"Thank God for that. I would not want to be married to a wimpette anyway."

"Count your blessings, Michael."

"Father, here we are. This is where I stay. These apartments are all owned by the hospital. Residents and fellows who are not married may live here. I have a one-bedroom apartment. Actually, they are just like one-bedroom hotel rooms except that they have a kitchen and sink."

When they entered Michael's apartment, Father John said, "This is a pretty spacious room."

"I am going to move out of this apartment when we get back from Hawaii."

"Do you have your two-bedroom apartment ready?"

"It is livable. We just have to decorate it when we get back from our honeymoon."

"I see."

"Father John, you can stay in the apartment while we are in Hawaii."

"Michael, I have to get back to Indiana as soon as possible. I want to leave after the wedding dinner. My assistant is sick. I have to hear confessions on Saturday afternoon. I hope you and Laura will understand."

"We do. We are just so happy you could come and officiate at our wedding."

"Your wedding is very important to me. I raised you as a father should raise a son. I would feel very badly if I could not witness another milestone in your life. I owe it to you."

"Thank you, Father John. I know I can always count on you. You must be very tired. Why don't you take your shower now, so that you can sleep late tomorrow?"

"I will do that, Michael."

While Father John was taking a shower, Michael looked all through his journals for Charlie Singleton's letters. No luck. He could not remember where he had put them.

"I must find those letters," he mused. "There might be some secrets in them. They could explain things."

Michael heard Father John come out of the shower, "Father John, do you want some warm milk before you go to sleep?"

"No, thank you, Michael. I usually read the bible before I go to bed."

"Father, I am going to the hospital early. Do you want me to cook breakfast for you before I leave?"

"Thank you, Michael, but I can help myself."

"Do you want to read any particular book, Father?"

"No, I would like to go downtown and see the cathedral. Just tell me how to get the bus."

"I will give you a map of the city."

"That will be fine. Good night, Michael."

"Good night, Father John."

Michael was already gone when Father John woke up in the morning. He turned on the television station. A lawyer named Robert Smith was being interviewed on the news. He was being questioned about his candidacy for municipal judge.

"Do you think you would be able to perform the duties of a judge without being prejudiced by all your business dealings?"

"What business dealings? I resent the tone of your questions. Are you trying to imply I have a conflict of interest?"

"I am not implying," said the interviewer. "I am asking you a direct question."

Robert Smith walked out of the interview.

Father John took bus 159 to Center City. He got off at 15th and Chestnut St. and walked towards the cathedral. He went to the main entrance, but it was locked. So, he decided to walk towards Logan Square to the Art Museum. The Art Museum was also locked. He looked for a public phone, but all the phones were not working. He walked towards Chestnut St. to Spruce St.. Center City was crowded. He went towards Broad Street. He could see women and young children walking around with their dirty baggage.

"Is this the city of Brotherly Love? How come there are so many kids roaming around the streets with no food to eat and no place to call their home?" Father John asked himself.

He watched the kids walking behind their mothers. Pangs of sadness overcame him. Tears welled up in his eyes. "How sad and inhumane," said Father John to himself.

It was almost three o'clock when Father John arrived at Michael's apartment. He noticed that Michael's answering machine was blinking red. He rewound the tape. There was a message.

"Father John, I will be home by five o'clock. Please be ready; Mrs. Secula is inviting us to dinner. We are also going to St. Archangel's Church so that you will meet the pastor of the parish. Please help yourself to whatever food is in the frigidaire."

Father John looked out the window. The same scene that he saw downtown was being replayed in the busy intersection of University City. Kids were throwing darts and stones at each other. He had never seen so many fights in the street. He could really appreciate what he had left behind in Indiana. What a difference between city and rural life!

Michael arrived at exactly five o'clock.

"Father John, let's go. I want to show you around Independence Square. I want to show you where Edgar Allan Poe used to live. We can also pass by the house where Betsy Ross used to live. I wish I could drive you to Winterthur Museum at Brandywine, but we are too short of time."

"Don't worry, Michael. I will be coming back to visit you and Laura sometime in the future."

By six o'clock, Michael and Father John were already at the Secula residence. Dinner was being prepared by Mrs. Secula and Jeanie.

"Our appointment with the pastor of St. Archangel's Church is at seven o'clock. I don't mean to rush dinner, but that was the only slot available for Father Walls to see us."

"At least he was kind enough to squeeze us in his schedule since we were kind of late in notifying him."

"I know!"

"Mom, are you coming with us?"

"Yes, I think it would be a good idea for us to come with you."

"Jeanie, don't worry about the dishes. We will finish that in no time when we get back."

"No problem."

The five of them were at the rectory at the stroke of seven.

Mrs. Secula introduced everyone to Father Walls. Father Walls and Father John talked about how the ceremony would be conducted. The dress rehearsal would be in two days. Father Walls gave them permission to use special pots with fresh flowers and wide white ribbons. Laura's Uncle Joseph would be giving her away.

The five of them went back to the Secula residence.

"Does anyone care to have something to drink?" asked Mrs. Secula.

"No, thank you," responded Father John. "Michael and I have to go back early. I want Michael to show me around Center City tonight before we head home to his apartment."

"I will be glad to show you around Center City, Father."

Michael and Father John said good night to the Seculas.

"Michael, why are you taking a different route?"

"We are going to drop by St. John Neumann's chapel. I am sure the church doors are not locked yet. We can also go through the rectory if the church doors are already locked."

"I hear that a lot of people go on pilgrimages there."

"Yes, it is true. I have also read about a young boy with Reye's Syndrome who was miraculously cured by St. John Neumann."

"I have read about that miracle, too."

Father John and Michael parked in front of the church.

The church doors were already locked. The rectory doors were also locked.

"Do you want to knock, Father John?"

"No, probably the Fathers are resting now. I will have a chance to visit this church sometime in the future."

"I will take you downtown now. Why the interest in downtown, Father?"

"I want to survey the number of homeless people that sleep on the sidewalk. I would like to have an idea of the number of women and children."

"Father John, the children and their mothers usually sleep in empty buildings which they have to vacate during the day. Homeless men usually sleep on the sidewalk near the vents to keep themselves warm. Sometimes they use newspapers to keep themselves warm."

"How sad. I never saw so much poverty and hunger until I arrived here."

"Father John, you must realize that this is inner city Philadelphia. Some of these people are here because they are down on their luck. Some of them have lost their jobs, and eventually their houses were foreclosed. They have no place to go, their self-esteem is drained, and they have no relatives to help them. They end up in the street trying to survive by panhandling and scavenging for food. Some of them are drug addicts, alcoholics, or mentally ill whose families are afraid to take care of them because they are unmanageable. Some of them are just plain unfortunate and have been evicted from their apartments because they are unemployed and can't afford to pay the rent."

"The city needs to find houses to shelter all these people."

"I agree with you, Father John. The city could ask for volunteers to rehabilitate all the abandoned houses for the homeless. But, there is a lot of resistance from the community. People are afraid to have former homeless people as neighbors. They are afraid the value of their property will go down."

"But unfortunate people should really mingle with the rest of the community to learn how other people manage to survive their own misfortunes."

Michael was driving along Chestnut St. when they heard a police siren. Apparently, there had been some shooting in an apartment due to domestic violence. Michael parked his car at the sidewalk and watched the estranged husband being arrested.

"Michael, it is not only homeless people that you worry about when you live in the city. You have to worry about muggers and pickpockets, too."

"Father John, I am very careful when I go downtown, even during the day. I have read about crimes being committed in broad daylight, too. There is really no safe place to live anymore. Philadelphia needs more policemen to protect each citizen."

"I could not agree more."

"We are here now. I am not going to the hospital tomorrow. We will have our dress rehearsal at six in the evening. Dinner will be at eight at the Secula residence."

By five-thirty in the evening the next day, Michael and Father John were at the Secula residence. The five of them went to St. Archangel's Church and met the rest of the bridal entourage there. The dress rehearsal went very well. The organ player was there, too. She played Wagner's "Ave Maria." After the dress rehearsal, everyone went to the Secula residence where dinner was served. Michael and Father John left by ten o'clock. They did not arrive at Michael's apartment until eleven-thirty because of traffic on the Schuylkill Expressway. A tractor trailer had overturned, and the road was filled with sand, gravel and stones. Traffic had to be detoured. Michael ended up taking Ridge Ave. to City Line. They were both so exhausted when they got home, they both fell asleep soundly.

CHAPTER XXII

March 17, 1984, was Laura Secula and Michael Olsire's big day. Laura woke up early for her appointment at the beauty parlor. Her mom and Jeanie were coming with her. Her relatives from South Philadelphia were starting to arrive. Every one of them was excited for her. She was the first cousin to get married. There would be no flower girl or ring bearer, but it was going to be a traditional Italian wedding.

Michael called Laura.

"Father John and I are going to the barbershop. What time do we have to be at the church?"

"Five-thirty. The processional will be at exactly six o'clock. You have to be there ahead of the bridal entourage."

"I understand. We will be there on time. We will see you at church."

In the meantime, at the university hospital, the sheriff walked up to the information desk.

"Where can I get in touch with the following doctors: Jay Simmons, James Dillon, Michael Olsire, and John Miller?"

"Dr. Simmons has retired; Dr. Dillon has finished his fellowship. Dr. Olsire is on vacation, and Dr. Miller is only available for emergency situations."

"How come?"

"He is going to Dr. Olsire's wedding."

"Do you know where the reception is going to be held?"

"I don't know. Why are you asking me all these questions?"

"I have been trying to deliver these summons to these doctors for the last twenty-nine days, but, everytime I came here, I was told that they were either in surgery, not available, or on vacation. This is the last day I can deliver these summons. Otherwise, the complaint has to be refiled."

"Well, don't tell me that you will deliver these summons today!"

"I will try to."

"It will be very cruel of you to do that today."

"I am just doing my job."

"You are going to cause much grief and unhappiness if you persist."

"Everyone has to do what is expected of him."

"I am not going to tell you where the reception will be held."

"I have ample time to find out before twelve midnight."

"You are a pest. Please leave before I call the security guard."

"You don't have to. I have gotten enough information from you to work on. I assure you, these summons will be delivered tonight."

At St. Archangel's Church, Father John, Michael, and James Dillon had arrived by five-thirty. They looked over the church decorations. Every flower pot and ribbon was perfectly placed near each pew. The organist had already arrived and was trying to go over the processional song which she was going to play. The guests were starting to arrive at the church slowly and quietly. They were ushered in by John Miller. The Simmonses and the Cortezes, Michael's residents, and Laura's co-residents had arrived, too. The crowd was expecting the arrival of Laura anytime now.

The bridal party arrived in a black limousine. Laura's Uncle Joseph was seated in the front seat of the limousine. Laura, Jeanie, and Mrs. Secula were seated in the back. The bridal entourage was now ready to march down the aisle. Michael and James Dillon positioned themselves at the foot of the altar. The wedding entourage started walking down the aisle to the tune of "Ave Maria." All the guests stood up, trying to get a glimpse of the lovely bride.

As soon as Laura and her uncle reached the foot of the altar, Michael shook hands with Joseph and, taking Laura's hand, walked with her slowly towards Father John whose eyes were solemnly fixed on the couple.

Laura and Michael both knelt on the pew at the center of the altar.

Father John said the mass and conducted the marriage ceremony which lasted about forty-five minutes. The Communion part took longer than usual because most of the guests received Holy Communion.

Everyone stood up after the wedding ceremony to get a glimpse of the bride and groom as they were about to leave the church and get into the bridal limousine.

The photographer, who had already taken pictures of the bride and her family, was on his way to the reception hall so he could be ready to take more pictures.

Father John rode with the bridal party. After they arrived at Sorrento, the reception line's picture was taken. The video camera was positioned in such a way that the guests' pictures could be taken as they passed through the reception line.

Everyone was taken with Laura's elegance and beauty. She was poised and radiant. Michael and Laura were very happy. The guests were all finally seated by seven o'clock. There were appetizers and an open bar. The bridal party occupied the slightly elevated bridal table. A toast for the happiness of the bridal couple was made by James Dillon.

The waitresses started serving dinner. The band started playing music while everyone was eating. Halfway through dinner, Laura and Michael stood up to dance. Everyone then started dancing. Michael danced with Mrs. Secula, too. Everyone started dancing in groups to the tune of the "Alley Cat."

Laura threw her bouquet in front of all the gathered single girls. When Jeanie caught the bouquet, everyone clapped.

All of a sudden, there was silence as a towering, authoritative person entered the reception hall and called out the names of the four doctors. The four walked towards the guy. He made them sign papers and handed each one of them a summons.

"I am sorry to do this to you tonight. I have been trying to deliver these summons for thirty days now. You were never around in the hospital whenever I came. You left me no choice but to deliver them tonight. Tonight is the thirty-day deadline for delivery. Otherwise, the complaint has to be refiled."

The four doctors were stunned. They decided to go to the men's room to read the summons.

The summons all contained the same complaint: Patricia Singleton and daughters, Kathleen and Michelle, were suing the four doctors for the wrongful death of Charles Singleton due to negligent infliction of the AIDS virus. Jury trial was demanded.

"My God, how can Patty do this to us? I myself am worried about getting AIDS because I accidentally was cut by a knife during his second surgery. This is such an injustice!"

"I don't know what to say. I did not even talk to or touch this patient in the accident ward."

"I feel so badly for all of you. The plaintiff lawyer will never see me because we are flying to Ireland in a couple of days."

"Will this summons affect my move to Ohio?"

"I don't think so, John. We have to call the insurance company to see what the lawyer says."

"Michael, you look so pale and exhausted. Are you alright?"

"I don't feel well. I am very hurt by Patty's false accusation. I thought I did more than my best. I thought she appreciated my kindness and concern for the whole family. I thought she really meant it when she said many times that I was a very caring doctor."

"You cannot trust patients all the time. As soon as they meet an unethical lawyer and are hard up for money, they forget what kindness and gratitude mean. They listen to the lawyer while he builds up his case so he can intimidate a physician into settling a frivolous suit."

"I wonder if this Robert Smith had an expert review the chart before he filed the lawsuit?"

"We will find out soon."

"Michael, relax. This is your wedding day. It could be worse. The plaintiff lawyer has to prove negligence beyond a reasonable doubt before he can win this case."

"I hope you are right."

"Let's go back to the wedding hall and dance."

"It's almost eleven o'clock. Father John has to be driven back to the airport. His plane leaves at 12:05 a.m."

"I will take care of that," said John Miller.

"Thank you, John."

"You are welcome, Michael."

Michael did not know what to do. Should he tell Laura now or later? He decided not to tell her.

"What's wrong, Michael? Why are you in such a pensive mood? It seems like the whole world has fallen on your shoulders."

"I am just a little tired."

"Do you want something to drink?"

"No."

"Well, let's go and dance then."

"Whatever you say."

"Why don't you dance with Debbie? I am going to ask Dr. Simmons to dance with me."

"That would be fine."

They approached Dr. Simmons and his daughter.

"Dr. Simmons, I would like to dance with you."

"It would be my pleasure, Laura."

As they moved onto the dance floor, Laura asked, "Dr. Simmons, I would like to ask you a personal question if you don't mind."

"What is it, Laura?"

"We all saw that man hand papers to you, Michael, James, and John. What is it all about?"

"Laura, we will discuss that later on, as soon as all the guests are gone. I can't tell you now. It is something very serious, and it concerns our medical careers. Michael was quite shocked tonight. So, be patient with him. He is devastated. He has been betrayed by his friends."

"I can't understand this."

"You will, later on. Let's change the topic of conversation. Let's go back to our table. You and Debbie and the rest of your friends can exchange pleasantries. Debbie is excited about her job as an assistant medical examiner. She is looking forward to it. She wants to take criminology classes at night."

"That would really help her when she does forensic pathology."

"I would hope so."

The guests started to leave by 12:30 a.m. John Miller, who had taken Father John to the airport, had not come back yet. By 1:00 a.m., when all the guests were gone, John Miller finally arrived. Father John was on his way to South Bend, Indiana.

Laura and Debbie went to the hotel room that they had reserved to get changed. Michael and Laura were supposed to stay in the hotel tonight and leave early in the morning for Hawaii.

"I don't think we should go to Hawaii if Michael is this upset."

"Why is Michael upset?"

"I don't know. We will find out later on."

Laura and Debbie dolled themselves up before they went downstairs.

"Laura, Debbie, sit over here."

"What is this all about?"

"Laura, brace yourself. Don't get upset."

"Upset about what?"

"Do you remember Patty Singleton?"

"Of course I do."

"Well, she is suing all of us for medical negligence."

"On what grounds?"

"We don't know yet. This is just a notice that we are being sued. The complaints will be filed later."

"So, what are you going to do now?"

"We have to call our insurance carrier. The hospital is being sued, too."

"I don't know what to say."

"This is terrible."

"Charlie Singleton was operated on as an emergency; we had no choice but to give him blood. Otherwise, the anesthesiologist would not have administered anaesthesia."

"Is this the payoff you get for saving somebody's life?" asked Debbie.

"This is so unjust. There are a lot of doctors who commit medical malpractice and get away with it, but suing a doctor for caring and saving someone's life is just unconscionable."

"It is insane."

"It has to be stopped."

"Greedy, unethical lawyers should be stopped."

"This Robert Smith should be disbarred. I wonder if he is the same Robert Smith with a red birthmark at the nape of his neck."

"Why did you say that, Michael?"

"I don't remember. Someone told me about a Robert Smith with a red birthmark like that. I think it might have been Charlie."

"For God's sake, please try to remember who told you."

"I will."

"Well, it's now five o'clock in the morning. We better go home."

"Michael, call me before you leave for Hawaii."

"I will do that, Dr. Simmons."

Laura and Michael went up to their room. All of sudden, Michael collapsed in the bathroom.

Laura quickly dialed the hotel operator for an ambulance. Michael's pulse was good, although it was quite high at 98/min.

"Michael, Michael! Can you hear me?"

"Yes, Laura."

"What do you feel?"

"I have this terrible crampy pain. I feel like I am going to pass out again."

"Please, don't do this to me!"

Laura could hear the ambulance siren coming closer. The ambulance paramedics rushed to their room.

"Over here please. Where are you going to take us?"

"The closest hospital is Smithsvale Hospital."

"Please, can't you take us to University Hospital?"

"No, we have to abide by regulations. We have to take you to the closest hospital."

Laura stayed with Michael in the ambulance. Smithsvale Hospital accident ward was packed. There had just been a head-on collision nearby, and two passengers had been pronounced dead.

Laura was familiar with some of the medical staff. She called Dr. Reeves.

Dr. Reeves responded immediately since he was in the accident ward admitting an elderly patient in severe heart failure.

"Thank you, Dr. Reeves, for coming in immediately."

"Young lady, how can I ever forget you? I learned a lot of pearls from you about Acute Disseminated Necrotizing Fasciitis. L-tryptophan causes a variant of Acute Disseminated Necrotizing Fasciitis and is known as Eosinophilia Myalgia Syndrome. Do you realize that twenty-three people have already died from taking L-tryptophan?"

"I have read about it, Dr. Reeves. This young man is my husband. We were married today. But, unfortunately, our festivities were marred by a medical malpractice summons."

"How cruel!"

"What do you think is wrong with Michael?"

"I don't know yet. Michael describes his major symptom as a crampy abdominal pain. He says that he feels like his intestines are being squeezed and stretched."

"I hope it is not Crohn's Disease or Diverticulitis."

"I hope so, too. I am going to start intravenous fluids with vitamins. We will draw all the blood tests, and then I will do a CAT Scan as soon as he can tolerate oral feedings. I definitely do not think that this is food poisoning."

"Thank you, Dr. Reeves. Would you please write on the order sheet that I am allowed to stay with him?"

"I will do that. Please don't hesitate to call me if you feel Michael's condition changes. You will be acting as his personal physician."

"I hope I don't miss anything since I am so emotionally involved."

"I will see you later on."

"Thank you, Dr. Reeves."

Michael was finally transferred to a single room on the medical floor. Laura called her mom and Jeanie for them to come to the hospital.

"What's wrong with Michael?"

"Michael collapsed in the bathroom of our hotel. He has severe abdominal pain. He has no vomiting or diarrhea. He just collapsed."

"We will be there shortly. Do you need anything?"

"Michael needs some clothes and a robe. I need some clothes, too. The nursing director will probably let me take a shower in one of the call rooms. I will give you the keys to our apartment. Don't rush. Michael is asleep. Dr. Reeves gave him a Demerol injection for pain relief. I will see you later. I will have to go down to the cafeteria to get something to eat. Bye."

Laura was still eating in the cafeteria when Mrs. Secula and Jeanie had her paged. She hugged her mom and Jeanie and then started crying!

"I hope nothing is wrong with Michael. I hope he is just exhausted. We did not go up to our room until five o'clock in the morning."

"How come?"

"Because all of them were very upset."

"Who is 'them'?"

"Dr. Simmons, Michael, James Dillon, and John Miller. They are all being sued by Patty Singleton and her daughters for medical malpractice."

"For goodness sake! What is wrong with these people?"

"Michael gave of himself to them. What more do they want from him?"

"His blood and money, I guess. Suing doctors is better than winning a lottery ticket. It is tax-free, unless it is for punitive damage."

"Well, I am sure Patty is going to lose. This lawyer must be unethical and greedy!" exclaimed Jeanie.

Laura said, "Dr. Simmons, who did not even examine, touch, or talk to the patient, is being sued, too. This doctor has devoted his whole life to taking care of his patients and to teaching and training residents all over the world, and this is what he gets in his retirement. It is so unfair!"

"Laura, don't get yourself upset. You have to show Michael that you are strong. You could be in Michael's situation, too."

"Mom is right, Laura. Every patient is a potential plaintiff."

"I know. But, of all people, Patty and her daughters! Mrs. Collins was right. Patty is up to no good. I think Mrs. Collins was trying to tell us something when Michael and I visited her in the nursing home."

By the next morning, Michael's crampy pain had subsided. Dr. Reeves saw him and was very optimistic. He requested a consult with a gastroenterologist after the CAT Scan came back normal. The colonoscopy showed only Irritable Bowel Syndrome.

Both Laura and Michael were jubilant to hear the good news. Michael would be discharged within the next two days, as soon as all his electrolytes became normal.

Jeanie and Mrs. Secula had already gotten Laura and Michael's luggage from the hotel. They also cleaned the apartment and bought some food for them. They also put up the drapes and did all the wash. Laura and Michael, however, would have to add finishing touches to the apartment's decor.

On March 21, 1984, Michael was discharged from the hospital. He still looked haggard, but he preferred to be home rather than to spend another restless night on a hospital bed.

"Michael, you still look tired and pale."

"I know, but I would rather sleep and rest in the apartment."

"I have to make you chicken soup when we get home."

"That would be fine. I don't know why I feel so exhausted."

"You have every reason to be exhausted from stress. I would be, too, if I got a summons that I was being sued by people who I thought were my friends. I would be very hurt and probably depressed and unable to eat for a couple of days."

"I am glad you understand what I am going through. At least, I have you to listen and share my grief and pain."

"I can understand your situation. I could be in the same predicament as you. But, let us not talk about this supposed malpractice. There was no malpractice committed here. You have nothing to do with Charlie's AIDS. It was drug induced. But, we have no way of proving it. At that time, in Charlie's case, we were dealing with a legal powerhouse. I am almost positive this guy had connections in high places and with a drug cartel. How could he supply all those drugs to the homeless downtown? Is he connected with the cops? Where does he live? Does he have kids selling drugs in the street? Is he the same Robert Smith who is suing you? We have to find answers to all these questions. We need to do the detective work fast, before your case goes on trial."

"Dr. Simmons has already sent a copy of the chart to the insurance company and to the defense lawyer. Now we have to wait for the formal complaints and interrogatories. Dr. Simmons is also getting copies of all the charts of the homeless patients who died of AIDS. So far, he has found eight patients. Two of these patients died before Charlie was even admitted to the university hospital. We have to check all the connections of these homeless patients."

"I will call Debbie tonight to see what I can do to help. Probably, I can also check the list of AIDS patients at Northend Hospital and find out where they used to hang out."

"Be careful, Laura. I don't want you to jeopardize your residency, even though I want to win this case."

"I will. Don't worry. I will just ask the other residents about possible AIDS patients whom they have treated or who have died in the hospital the past two years."

"Laura, you better get some sleep. I hope you don't get tired taking care of me."

"Just get well before I go back to work on Monday so that I don't have to worry about you while I am operating."

Michael finally fell asleep. Laura tiptoed to the next room and tried to go over Michael's journals and books one by one. She could not find what she was looking for. She went through all the boxes that Michael had accumulated throughout his residency - no luck! She went through Michael's clothes, coats, towels, and sheets, still no luck! She looked over the florigraphy books of Michael. Finally, she found the florigraphy book, "Laura," that Michael had given her on Valentine's Day. There were two sealed letters addressed to Michael, both of which were not to be opened until two years after Charlie's death.

"My God, what should I do with these letters? Should I tell Michael to open them now?"

Laura took the two letters out of the florigraphy book and placed them on the table.

She fell asleep on the sofa instead of going back to their bedroom. She did not want to wake up Michael, who, for the first time, was having a restful sleep in a quiet and peaceful surrounding.

CHAPTER XXIII

Laura left for work early Monday morning. Michael was still sleeping peacefully. She left him a note on the table.

As soon as Laura got to the hospital, the telephone operator paged all the surgical residents to go to the trauma center immediately. There had been a serious head-on collision in front of the university. Three people were brought in DOA. Another patient was a young lady whose pretty face had been disfigured by multiple bone fractures of the face. She was the youngest daughter of the chief pathologist. Her eyes were black and blue. The whites of her eyes had been replaced by blood clots. She could hardly breathe without experiencing severe chest pain. She had about seven fractured ribs as shown on a chest X-Ray. Her abdomen was rigid as a board due to ruptured organs. The bedside abdominal tap was positive for blood. The X-Ray of her pelvis and extremities showed multiple broken bones and a fractured right leg. A Mast Trouser was applied temporarily to stop the bleeding.

Laura called the thoracic surgeon, the general surgeon and an orthopedic surgeon. The anaesthologist did an awake intubation. There were about twenty-five doctors attending to this patient. She was wheeled immediately to the operating room.

The patient kept asking Laura before she was intubated, "Am I going to be disfigured? Am I going to have a scar on my face?"

Laura squeezed the patient's hand and said in a very low voice, "Let's hope not."

Laura was fighting back her emotions. She knew deep down that she had lied to the patient. How could she tell her that she should not worry about a disfigured face, but about her survival? The sight of a young, pretty woman almost on a gruesome deathbed practically ripped apart Laura's emotional bearings.

Everyone was busy trying to keep the vital signs of the patient stable. On opening the abdomen, the surgeon saw about 3500 cc of blood. The liver, spleen, and inferior vena cana were all lacerated. Blood was suctioned; the aorta was tamponaded. A splenectomy was done, the inferior vena cana was repaired, and the liver was mobilized and packed. Two attending surgeons did all the abdominal operations with Laura and the senior surgical resident.

O negative blood was continuously being pumped.

The thoracic surgeon opened the left and right chest wall. But, suddenly, the patient's heart stopped! A young lady had become lifeless and a part of a statistic due to a fatal car accident. A young lady had been robbed of life, robbed of an opportunity to go to college, robbed of an opportunity to be married, and robbed of an opportunity to have children of her own!

Such a ghastly medical emergency left feelings of sadness, grief, and visceral emptiness in the caring physicians, and they were reminded again that they couldn't save everyone, but that they could help in the emotional healing of the grieving family.

Everyone who was involved in the efforts to save this lady's life went to talk to her father. What, though, do you tell a colleague? Do you tell him that you have failed to save his daughter's life? Or, do you tell him you are sorry and sit down and cry with him?

Laura sat down and cried with the couple. She could empathize with them. All she had to think about was the sudden death of her father and the kindly gestures and thoughtfulness that Michael showed them while they were still in shock.

"Would you care to have coffee?"

"No, thank you. You are very kind," said the grieving Mrs. Van Weese.

"I have to go back to work now, Mrs. Van Weese. If there is anything I can do for you, please page me."

"We will. Thank you."

Laura was physically and emotionally drained. She went up to her room to rest for thirty minutes before her surgical clinic started. She was reading the *Philadelphia Gazette* obituary section when she noticed: "Ann Collins, 75-year-old, beloved mother of Patricia Singleton, died peacefully at Bellwood Nursing Home. Viewing and funeral services Saturday morning. No flowers."

Laura immediately called Michael.

"Mrs. Collins died two days ago. The viewing and funeral will be on Saturday."

"Poor lady! Why do you think it's taking this long for the burial?"

"The nursing home probably had a hard time locating Patty."

"It's a shame; she died with bad feelings for Patty."

"You can't blame Mrs. Collins. She would have been more upset if she had known about the lawsuit Patty filed against the four of you."

"I know, but we should not condemn Patty because we don't really know what is going on in her mind."

"How can you be so charitable, Michael? She has already stabbed you in the back."

"But this is not the real Patty I know. Euridis, who seems to be always with her, makes me suspicious."

"I hope you are right, Michael. By the way, did you see the two sealed letters on the table?"

"Yes, I did. Those letters are going to stay sealed."

"Michael, please open them up. Your career is hanging in the balance. I am sure these letters will help you somehow, or Charlie would not have written them before he died."

"Laura, it would be intellectually dishonest to do that."

"I am sorry for even asking you to open them up. You are such an honest man."

"Thank you. It always pays to be honest."

"Are we going to go to the viewing and funeral?"

"I think so. We have to. Mrs. Collins was always nice to us."

On Saturday, Michael and Laura went to Miraculous Medal Church early. Patty and her daughters were seated in the first pew. Michael and Laura greeted the three of them. Patty was surprised to see them. She was speechless!

"How did you find out about Mom's death, Dr. Olsire?"

"Laura read it in the *Philadelphia Gazette* obituary."

"Thank you for coming to pay your last respects to Mom."

"You are welcome, Patty."

The funeral mass was said by Father O'Keefe who had known Ann Collins since kindergarten. He also said the eulogy. Mrs. Collins was buried at Holy Sepulchre Cemetery in the same plot where her husband was buried.

After the funeral, Michael and Laura bade goodbye to Patty and her daughters.

"I know you feel uncomfortable with me. It is not what you think. I filed that lawsuit not for money, but for justice."

"I did not do any injustice to Charlie. I did more than my best in taking care of him."

"Dr. Olsire, someday you will understand why I am doing what I am doing now."

"You have caused my husband a lot of grief and pain. Is this what he gets for caring too much?"

"Someday you will understand, Dr. Secula."

"I hope that day comes soon."

"Well, Patty, Michelle, and Kathy, we have to go now."

"Thank you for your kindness to Grandmom," Michelle and Kathy said in unison.

"You are welcome." Laura and Michael left.

"Mom, how could you sue Dr. Olsire? He is the only friend we have."

"You don't know the whole story, and I can't tell you. You will find out sooner or later."

"Why can't you tell us, Mom? We are the only family you have left."

"I can't because there are other people involved. This is a very critical situation."

"What do you mean by 'critical'?"

"Please, do not ask me too many questions. Let us keep this topic out of our conversation for good."

"But, Mom, we are concerned about Dr. Olsire. He has been good to us. He is our friend. I think this has affected him. He was kind of aloof to us."

"Trust me. This lawsuit has nothing to do with Dr. Olsire personally."

"We hope so. It would be a terrible payback for all his kindnesses."

"I wish I could convince him without any explanation, but it would be very difficult for me to do that now. I just hope he will understand when the truth finally comes out."

"We hope so, too. We do not want to lose his friendship."

"I know, and I am sorry; this medical malpractice lawsuit has really strained it."

Laura dropped off Michael at their apartment. She had to go back to Northend Hospital to finish her charts, make rounds, and relieve Dr. Saltine.

Laura could not concentrate on doing her charts. She was too preoccupied with the things Patty had told them at the funeral. She finally decided to go up to her call room and rest. She fell asleep while she was reading her surgical journal.

Laura was awakened at around nine-thirty in the evening by the nurse from the accident ward. An elderly woman had just been brought in to the accident ward with a stab wound on her abdomen. She was not shocky, but her abdomen was very distended with muscle guarding. The suspect had not been arrested yet. Laura went down immediately to the emergency room.

"Let us get all the blood testing and type and cross of blood immediately. Get a STAT CAT Scan, too. I will call the attending so that he can come and scrub with me. Is there anyone with this lady?"

"The police car left to get her daughter. They should be in shortly. The lady lives by herself. The suspect is a teenager who lives in the neighborhood. He is on drugs. According to the police, there was no forced entry in her house. He used to run errands for this lady."

"It's a shame. Some of these kids have no respect for the elderly. It is like stabbing his own grandmother."

The patient, Mrs. Martin, was immediately prepared for exploratory laparotomy. STAT CAT Scan showed some evidence of bowel rupture in that area of the cul de sac. As soon as the attending physician, Dr. Reighler, came in, Mrs. Martin was ready to be wheeled down to the operating room. A crash induction was done. Her daughter arrived after her mother had been wheeled down to the operating room.

The abdomen was opened, and fecal matter was noted all over the cul de sac; this was suctioned and removed piecemeal with laparotomy sponges. A diversion colostomy was done, and the patient was put on massive antibiotic therapy. The patient was going to be moved to the ICU for monitoring. Laura thanked everyone and rushed outside to talk to the daughter of Mrs. Martin.

"I am Dr. Secula. I helped operate on your Mom. Whatever knife the assailant used cut through her large intestines. We had to do a colostomy. She is on the critical list. We also have her on massive antibiotics. Let's keep our fingers crossed and hope for the best. You may stay with her and, if you have any more questions, please feel free to call me. I will be around. I have to go back to the recovery room to write some orders. You can walk down with me if you want. I will let you into the recovery room since there are only a few people around there now."

"Thank you, Dr. Secula. I have to make some phone calls. I will meet you in the ICU."

Laura went back to the recovery room. She noticed that the Foley Catheter was empty.

"Cindy, how much urine did you measure from the Foley Catheter?"

"Ten cc."

"We have to hydrate her more, and I will call a medical consultation. I have to put in a central line to monitor her intake and output. We have to watch her closely. Please get a STAT CBC, and I will call the laboratory for the gram stain of the abdominal culture we took. I might have to call the infectious disease fellow. I am afraid she might go into septic shock."

The medical resident came in and started the patient on rapid digitalization. Laura inserted the central line. The infectious disease fellow added another broad spectrum antibiotic.

Laura paged Donna Martin.

"Donna, I want you to come down to the recovery room. I have a lot of things to explain to you."

Donna came down immediately.

"Donna, I am sorry to tell you that your mom is not doing as well as I thought she would."

"What do you mean, Dr. Secula?"

"Your mom's urine output is quite low. I had to put in a central line. I called in the medical resident and the infectious disease fellow. They will help me take care of her. As soon as we get her stabilized, we will move her to the ICU. I think you better stick around. Have you eaten your dinner?"

"Not yet. I don't feel like eating now. I would rather wait here and go up with you to the ICU."

"That would be fine. Were you able to call all the people you wanted to call?"

"Not really."

"As soon as your mom is stabilized, I will let you call through the hospital line."

"Thank you, Dr. Secula."

"Dr. Secula, Dr. Henry thinks we can move Mrs. Martin to the ICU now."

"Let's go then."

Laura helped Cindy wheel Mrs. Martin to the ICU. Donna walked with them.

"Donna, please stay in the waiting room until we get your mom situated. I will call you as soon as it is feasible for you to see her."

"I will be waiting, Dr. Secula."

As soon as Mrs. Martin was moved from her stretcher, Laura took her pulse. It was 102.

"Please take the temperature of Mrs. Martin."

There was a pause and a silence.

"It is 95.6, Dr. Secula."

"Please get me 120 mg of Solu-Medrol and page the medical resident and the infectious disease fellow. I think Mrs. Martin is going into septic shock. Please get her daughter. I want her to see her mom before the situation becomes worse."

Donna was ushered into the room by the nurse. Laura held her hand tightly and took her aside.

"Donna, your mother has an overwhelming infection secondary to her lacerated large intestines. I am not sure whether she will make it. We are trying our best. I have given her Solu-Medrol. The medical resident and infectious disease fellow are also here trying to do their best. We gave her massive antibiotics in the operating room. We have to wait and see how she responds to all these medications."

Donna started crying. Laura put her hand around her shoulders and said, "I am sorry we can't do more for your mom. All the odds are against her because of her age and the overwhelming infection on an unprepared bowel. I will be back as soon as I can. Is there anything you want me to do for you?"

"Yes, please do not code my mother. Let her die in peace."

"I will put that on her chart. Is there anything else you want me to do for you?"

"Thank you, Dr. Secula. You have done more than enough. Just explaining to me what has transpired since my mother came to the hospital and taking the time to update me on her progress are more than enough. You have done your best. Everyone has been attentive to my mother. I cannot thank you enough for all your kindness."

"Don't be upset if you see the detectives here. This is going to be a case of homicide. The detectives will be in shortly to ask questions."

"I understand."

Laura went back to Mrs. Martin's room. Her respiration was labored, her urine output was practically nil. Her pulse was hardly palpable.

Laura went to get Donna Martin.

"Donna, I am sorry to tell you that your mom's kidneys are shot. There is nothing more we can do for her."

"I understand. May I see her before she closes her eyes?"

"Yes, you may. She is in a coma."

Laura went inside Mrs. Martin's room with Donna. The nurse who was taking care of her could not get the heartbeat anymore. The electrocardiogram had a flat tracing. Mrs. Martin just succumbed. Laura looked at Donna Martin's shocked expression. Laura herself was overwhelmed by feelings of sadness and helplessness. "We can't save everyone's life, no matter how hard we try. We are only human," she thought.

Laura took Donna to an empty room.

"Donna, please cry. Do not hold back your tears. Everything is in the hands of God now."

"Dr. Secula, Dr. Secula, " a voice on the loudspeaker interrupted.

"Excuse me, someone is paging me. Hello, yes, I am Dr. Secula. I will be there as soon as I can. Donna, the detectives are here. Please come with me. They want to ask you questions, too."

The two women went out to the nurses' station.

"Donna Martin, I am Detective Surefire. I would like to ask you a few questions. When was the last time you saw your mother?"

"One week ago."

"When was the last time you talked to her?"

"Two days before she was stabbed."

"Do you know who runs errands for her?"

"Yes, the boy across the street."

"What is his name?"

"David Sellick."

"How old is he?"

"I don't know."

"Would you be able to recognize him if you saw him?"

"I think so."

"We will have to do an autopsy on your mother, but you can make the funeral arrangement now. The funeral director will get in touch with the coroner's office. The autopsy report will not be back for two weeks to a month. The coroner's office is very busy," Laura told Donna.

"Dr. Secula, we will need a copy of Mrs. Martin's chart."

"I will have it xeroxed as soon as I can. Are you going to wait for it?"

"Yes. You have to get two copies. One for me, and one for the coroner's office."

"I will do that."

Donna Martin called Laura on Monday morning to thank her and to tell her that her mother's viewing would be on Tuesday evening.

"Thank you for telling me. My husband and I will try to be there. I will be off that day. Is there anything I can do for you?"

"No, thank you. You have done more than enough. I will see you at the viewing."

On Tuesday night, Michael and Laura attended Mrs. Martin's viewing. Laura noticed that even the detectives who came to the hospital were at the viewing. Laura just looked at them without saying anything. The viewing was crowded. Mrs. Martin had lived in that neighborhood for forty years. She had cultivated lots of friendships. Donna Martin thanked Michael and Laura for taking the time to come.

CHAPTER XXIV

On May 1st, 1984, Dr. Simmons and Michael received their interrogatories. They had to mail John Miller's and James Dillon's interrogatories to Ohio and Ireland respectively. The medical liability insurance company told them that, if John Miller and James Dillon did not answer the interrogatories and appear for the deposition when asked to, they would be disclaimed by the insurance company and would be liable for their judgements. Dr. Simmons called Dr. Dillon in Dublin.

"James, how are you doing?"

"I am fine, Dr. Simmons. What can I do for you?"

"Well, Michael and I just received the interrogatories for the Singleton case, and I mailed a copy for you to answer. Since you received the summons personally, you are obliged to answer these interrogatories and come back for the deposition when asked to. You have no choice. The medical liability insurance company may refuse to defend you if you don't answer the interrogatories and appear for the deposition."

"I just have to do it then. How is everyone there?"

"Michael is going to teach at the university as soon as he finishes his fellowship. Debbie and Laura are both fine. Jorge and Estela are doing well in their practice in Miami. John Miller's interrogatories were mailed to him. Michael called him this morning about the interrogatories. John is as upset as you are. What more can I say? If you come for the deposition, you are welcome to stay with us. Do you think you will bring your wife with you?"

"I do not know yet."

"Well, we will keep you informed of the progress of the litigation."

"Thank you, Dr. Simmons. Please give my love to everyone."

"I will do that."

Dr. Simmons and Michael got together to answer the interrogatories.

"These questions are ridiculous. It would take one hundred pages for me just to answer the questions about my credentials. This one question leaves me no choice but to do that."

"Dr. Simmons, the only question that really needs to be answered by you is about your credentials. You never examined or talked to Charlie Singleton. I will have to answer all these questions about Charlie's illness and my relationship with him."

"Well, we just have to give him a dose of his own medicine."

"We will see how our lawyer intends to defend us. We have to cooperate with him. This will be a test case in Pennsylvania. This is the first AIDS case that has been filed in Philadelphia."

"I hope we win. If the members of the jury are well informed about the disease, our chances of winning are high."

"I hope so."

"Michael, you have to be optimistic. This is not the end of the world. We should not let this greedy unethical lawyer intimidate us. He has no leg to stand on. I don't think he has a qualified expert to testify against us. I don't think he even asked an expert to review the chart before he filed the lawsuit."

"How can you know that?"

"Well, he requested the chart one week before he filed the lawsuit. The chart is about 3,000 pages long. There is no way he can convince me that a practicing physician would be able to go over the chart in that much time. He wouldn't be able to analyze the facts adequately and render an unbiased opinion, even if he were a speed reader."

"I could not agree more. Probably he has a hired gun who reviews medical charts regularly."

"You are probably right. Then, if that is the case, it will be easy to tear apart his credentials. Remember, Michael, that a medical malpractice case can be won or lost on the credentials of the expert."

"What do you mean?"

"How can this 'supposed' expert win a case if he has not seen or treated a patient with AIDS? The intelligence of the members of the jury should not be underestimated. They frown on these regular expert hired guns."

"Now I am beginning to understand more about the legal process."

"So, keep your fingers crossed. Don't get yourself too upset. It is not worth the stress you are putting yourself through. I bet you, if you got your cholesterol check now, it would probably be in the three hundred range."

"You are probably right, Dr. Simmons. We might as well finish answering the interrogatories now."

"Well, at least we do not have to answer all the irrelevant questions such as those on partnerships, termination of partnership, etc."

"This question about insurance coverage can be answered by our lawyer. He should have all this information from the insurance company."

"This question about the patient's condition at the time of treatment should be answered. The patient had a life-threatening condition that required immediate surgical intervention!"

"We do not have photographs of Charlie's surgical condition. I don't think this question is even relevant to his surgical condition."

"That question sounds so stupid."

"I agree with you. The first time he came to the accident ward, he was hypovolemic and shocky. What stupid doctor would waste his time taking photographs of a patient in this type of emergency situation? This question does not make sense."

"This question about the case being presented in both medical and surgical conferences is ridiculous."

"Yes, it was presented in both monthly medical and surgical conferences."

"Our lawyer can answer the questions about our expert witness and his credentials."

"I guess we have answered all the questions that we are supposed to answer."

"Our lawyer will fill in the rest. How is Laura doing?"

"Laura is doing well. Sometimes, I worry about her. She works too hard. She gets too emotionally involved with patients and their families. She always gets upset when something goes wrong with a patient, even if it is part of the course of the disease. I can tell as soon as she walks in our apartment how things went in the hospital."

"She will eventually learn to accept that she can't cure every patient, no matter how hard she tries."

"I hope so."

"Have a nice day, Michael. Keep in touch."

"Thank you, Dr. Simmons. Please say hello to Debbie for us. I hope she is enjoying her new job at the coroner's office."

"I certainly will."

CHAPTER XXV

Days, weeks, months went by. Laura and Michael continued to live the busy lives of surgical resident and surgical fellow. Laura was still moonlighting at Southern Hospital accident ward once a month. Michael was not quite keen about Laura's working in the accident ward. The accident ward coverage was the only sore spot in their relationship. But Laura had told Michael before they were married that she intended to do this to help out her widowed mother with ever-increasing real estate taxes and cost of utilities. Philadelphia was in such financial trouble that, every time the city needed money, the burden fell on the poor taxpayers.

It was August, 1984. Dr. Simmons and Michael had not heard anything from their lawyer. They presumed the ongoing litigation was progressing as it should.

On August 20, 1984, Laura was quite excited when she called Michael.

"Guess what, Michael?"

"What?"

"You are going to be a father soon."

"I am so delighted! When did you find out?"

"Today I had a quantitative beta subunits done. My hormone level is quite good, 9,000 MIU/ML. I did not tell you that I missed my period in August. I wanted to surprise you. Let's go and visit Mom and Jeanie tonight. I want them to share the good news with us."

"That would be nice. Are you going to come home first or do you want me to pick you up?"

"I think I want to come home first, and then you can do the driving."

"You are a mind reader. That was exactly what I was going to suggest."

"I will be home by five. I better hang up now. I want to do post-operative rounds before I leave."

"See you at five. Be careful driving and don't drive over many bumpy roads."

"Michael, you crack me up!"

As soon as Laura opened the door of the apartment, she noticed three red roses in a crystal vase and a card:

To my dear, lovely wife,
Thank you for the gift of life.
Love,
Michael

"Michael, where are you?"

"I am getting dressed. Did you see the three red roses on the table?"

"Yes, they are lovely!"

Michael came out of their room and hugged and kissed Laura.

"I am so happy! I have already called Father John to tell him that he would be a grandfather soon. He promised he would come up for the baby's christening."

"I would like to talk to him, too. We have to call him tonight as soon as we get back from Mom's."

"I am sure he would love to talk to you, too. He will probably give you a sermon on how you can stay healthy and carry a healthy baby."

"I still would like to tell him the good news myself. Let's get going, Michael, before the expressway gets crowded."

"We have to put the air conditioner on full blast. I don't want you to sweat too much. I don't want you to lose too much potassium and feel weak."

"Michael, I am fine. Our baby will be fine. I eat a well-balanced diet, and I was taking vitamins before I even got pregnant. I don't have any vices at all. So, what are you worried about?"

"I just want us to have a perfectly healthy child."

"So do I."

"What are we going to name our baby if it is a boy?"

"Well, if it is a baby boy, I would like to name him after you, Michael II. If it is a girl, I would like to name her Jennifer."

"Are you sure you want to name the baby Michael II if it is a boy?"

"I am positive. Michael is a very nice name. I would like him to grow up like his father."

"If it is a girl, we will name her Jennifer. I would like her to grow up like my wife."

"It is so uplifting to know that we have mutual admiration for each other."

"That's what marriage is all about."

"Here we are now. Mother is looking out the window."

Laura ran up the steps and hugged Mrs. Secula and Jeanie.

"Laura, be careful. You might fall!"

Laura, in her usual joking way, said to Michael, "Don't be a nervous father." To her mother she blurted, "Mom, you are going to be a grandmother soon!"

Mrs. Secula started sobbing.

"I am so happy for you and Michael. I wish your father were here. He would have been so happy! When is your delivery date?"

"Easter Sunday. I hope I go on time."

"You should have no problem. I had no problem with you and Jeanie. Let us have dinner now. I cooked your favorite meal, Veal Parmigiana."

"Mom, I am not going to have wine. Michael can have my wine. I am going to drive so Michael can enjoy his wine tonight. Also, pregnant women aren't supposed to drink alcoholic beverages."

"That is what I like about my wife! She is so considerate!"

"Naturally! I was raised by a nice and considerate mother. Jeanie, how come you are not talking?"

"I don't feel well today. There is so much going on in the office. There is a lot of people being laid off at work."

"Are you worried about your job?"

"No, but our company is relocating to New Jersey. I don't want to move there. I don't want to leave Mom by herself."

"Don't worry, Jeanie. You can always find another job. You are hard-working, and you have good credentials."

"Laura is right. You can always find another job with your skills."

"I hope so."

"Mom, Jeanie, it is getting late. We have to call Father John when we get home. I don't want to call him too late. He gets up very early for six o'clock mass. We will be back Saturday or Sunday depending on Michael's schedule."

Mrs. Secula and Jeanie walked Michael and Laura to the door.

"Be careful driving, Laura."

"I will, Mom."

Mrs. Secula and Jeanie kissed both Michael and Laura goodbye.

By the time they reached the expressway, Michael was already snoring.

"My poor husband must be very tired."

As soon as they arrived at the parking lot of their apartment, Laura woke up Michael.

"Michael, we are home now."

"Laura, why didn't you wake me up sooner?"

"You were very tired, Michael. I wanted you to get some extra sleep."

"I am so embarrassed. I let you do all the driving while I slept. Shame on me."

"Michael, please don't apologize. You are working too hard."

"Not as hard as you do."

"I know what you are trying to say. One more week, and I will give up my moonlighting job at Southern Hospital."

"Thank you, Laura. Now I don't have to worry about you every time you work in that bad neighborhood. Don't worry about Mom. We will help her out."

"Thank you, Michael."

As soon as they got into their apartment, Michael noticed that his books were all over the floor, but there was no sign of forcible entry. Michael looked over his florigraphy collection; they were all intact. Charlie's two letters were still there and still sealed.

"Michael, do you think someone tried to break into our apartment?"

"I don't know, Laura. There seems to be nothing missing."

"Should we report it to the police?"

"I don't know. Why don't you call Father John before it gets too late while I check to see if anything is missing in the apartment."

"I will do that. Don't you want to talk to him, too?"

"I will after you have talked to him."

Laura dialed Father John's number. Father John answered the phone himself.

"Father John, this is Laura. I am sorry I was not home when Michael called you. Did you hear the good news?"

"Yes, I am so delighted that I am going to be a grandfather soon. I've already started praying for you and the baby. Rest assured I will pray for a safe delivery for you. Michael is really on cloud nine. He was like a very happy little boy when he called today. How is your mom and Jeanie?"

"They are both fine and are both looking forward to the forthcoming blessed event. My due date is Easter Sunday, Father John. I hope the baby comes on time."

"Don't worry, Laura. Just pray to St. Gerard and the Miraculous Medal. Everything is going to be fine. Is Michael there?"

"He is here. I will get him for you. Take care of yourself, Father John, and we will be looking forward to seeing you at the baby's christening."

"I would not miss that for anything."

"Here's Michael, Father."

"I am so relieved, Father! Laura decided not to work in the accident ward anymore. I worry about her when she works at Northend Hospital, too. She has only one more year to go in her residency. Knowing Laura well, I am sure she would rather stay home and take care of the baby than operate the whole day. I don't want to tell her that. I want her to do it according to her own instinct."

"I agree with you, Michael. Laura is a very sensible lady. You are both very lucky to have each other.

Laura did very well with her pregnancy. She went to her obstetrician faithfully. She told her obstetrician she did not want an alpha-fetoprotein done (test for Spina Bifida). For her, it would not make any difference whether the alpha-fetoprotein was high or low. She did not want amniocentesis done either. She and Michael would love their child whether the child was perfect or deformed. They were both good practicing Catholics.

By her fourth month, Laura started having severe abdominal pain practically everyday. She had an ultrasound done which showed degenerating fibroid in the fundus of the uterus and a low-lying placenta. She had to take off from work and was placed on bedrest. She was also placed on home fetal monitoring because of her irritable uterus. The fetal monitor was checked twice a day at a central station by a nurse. Michael waited on her hand and foot. He would come home at lunch time to make her lunch. Before he left for work, Michael put Laura's breakfast by her bedside. Laura could not ask for a kinder and more thoughtful husband than Michael.

"Michael, I think you are pampering me. I will not know how to act after this baby is born. I am getting used to being served breakfast and lunch and dinner in bed!"

"Don't worry. As soon as the baby is born, you will be taking over the kitchen again. This is just a temporary arrangement."

"I will still have six weeks reprieve after the baby is born."

"I know that. Don't worry, I am a good house-husband! I will take off one week when you get home from the hospital."

"Mom will probably come here to help me take care of the baby during the first few weeks."

"I am sure she will."

Laura's abdominal pain came on and off the rest of her pregnancy. She decided to take a leave of absence. It had been difficult for her co-residents as well, but she knew her priority was her baby. Some of her co-residents, especially the males, resented her taking a long leave of absence. They had to take up the slack, so their moonlighting days in other hospitals had to be curtailed. This made Laura unpopular with the rest of the residents.

"Tough! My baby comes first."

"Laura, don't let your co-residents upset you. This is a typical macho reaction. I am sure that, if their wives had the same problem as you, they would feel the same way as I feel about you."

"I know, but I thought they were my friends!"

"Now you know they are not your friends. They are, at most, your acquaintances."

Laura left their apartment only for her obstetrical appointments. Michael always went with her and talked to Laura's obstetrician after each visit. Laura always took the last appointment slot so that other patients would not have to wait too long while Michael talked to her obstetrician.

Laura's pregnancy went along well. Even her weight gain had been within the normal range allowed in pregnancy. As her delivery time approached, her uterine irritability occurred more often. Her waddling gait was more pronounced. Her uterine measurements were progressively normal, but she felt as if the baby were too big for her pelvis. By her eighth month, she could hardly walk. Her pelvic bones hurt whenever she walked. She had to be put flat in bed, and a pelvic strap had to be put on her pelvic bones due to more-than-normal separation of the symphyseal bones. Laura was hoping that April would come soon. She started counting and marking the calendar every day. Finally, on April 13th, 1985, she started passing her mucous plug which was followed by bloody show.

At two in the morning of Easter Sunday, she went into active labor. Considering her inactivity for several months, Laura's labor was relatively short. It took her only nine hours for the cervix to be completely dilated and for the presenting part, the head, to come down the perineum.

Laura had local anaesthesia for her delivery. Michael was with her throughout her labor and delivery. At eleven o'clock in the morning, a healthy baby girl was delivered. Michael kissed Laura as soon as the baby girl was delivered. They both happily started crying. For Laura, though, these were not only tears of joy. She would be liberated from her five months of bed rest. She would have to practice to learn how to walk again.

The obstetrician took the baby to the crib under the light and suctioned mucus from her nasopharynx. The baby gave a lusty cry immediately after delivery. Her color was pink, and her respiration was good, as were her reflexes and muscle tone. The nurse handed the baby to Laura after cleaning off the vernix and wrapping her in a warm blanket.

"Jennifer has a good apgar. It is nine and ten. Laura has been a very good patient. I could not ask for a better patient."

"Dr. Kelvey, my wife followed your instructions to the letter."

"I can tell, and look at the big payoff, a beautiful, healthy little girl."

"Michael, I think Jennifer is a carbon copy of you! Just look at her blue eyes and curly black hair."

"Are you going to breastfeed, Dr. Secula?"

"I will."

Laura was wheeled back to the birthing room after her delivery. She had not wanted to deliver in the birthing room. She felt that, if a sudden complication had arisen, the proper equipment would have been more available in the delivery room. The rooms were bigger, too, in case more people needed to be called in. She was worried about infections, too. Since hospitals had relaxed the visiting regulations, too many people were able to walk in and out of the birthing rooms with only street clothes on. From Debbie's experience at the coroner's office, Laura found out that more women were dying postpartum because of infections. Or perhaps they were discharged too early, or perhaps vaginal cultures were not taken in order to cut cost (cost-containment). It was a shame that no hospital in the country released its infection rate to the public.

Laura was transferred to a private room on the regular maternity floor two hours after delivery.

As soon as Laura was transferred to her room, she called her mom and Jeanie. Her mom answered the phone.

"I was trying to call your apartment early this morning. I figured that when I did not get any answer you were probably enroute to the hospital. I was going to call the delivery room, but you beat me to it."

"Mom, you got your wish. Jennifer is here, and she weighs eight lbs. four oz. and is 23 cm. long. She looks like Michael. No trace of Secula traits at all."

"Well, as long she is healthy, that is all that matters. Jeanie and I will come and visit you after dinner. Is there anything you want me to bring?"

"Mom, I am so tired I would rather sleep than eat. Would you like to talk to Michael?"

"Please, put him on the phone."

When Laura put Michael on the phone, Mrs. Secula said, "Michael, I am so happy for you and Laura! Thank you for all your patience during Laura's pregnancy. It was hard on both of you."

"Everything is worth it. Once you see Jennifer, she will melt your heart. I am positive she will have a shiny and sweet disposition."

"Michael, do you want me to bring some food for you tonight?"

"Mom, I might not be here when you come. I have to go back to the hospital. Thanks for the thought. Do you want Laura again?"

"No, let her rest and sleep."

"Bye, Mom."

"Goodbye, Michael."

"Michael, you better go home and get some sleep before you go back to the hospital."

"I will, as soon as the nurse takes Jennifer. Laura, you have given me the gift of life. My life is so complete and fulfilled. God has been so good to me."

"We really have to count our blessings. We are both very lucky to have each other."

"We have to look forward to raising Jennifer. Raising kids nowadays is tough. There are so many distractions, including peer pressure."

"But, as long as we cultivate Jennifer's self-esteem, shower her with our love, and show her that we are good role models, I don't think she will have problems."

"I hope not."

"Michael, you must go home and rest now."

Michael kissed Laura and left.

Mrs. Secula and Jeanie visited in the evening. Mrs. Secula and Jeanie were ecstatic when they saw Jennifer.

"My God," said Mrs. Secula, "She looks exactly like Michael when he was an infant! She is so precious!"

"Laura, you know what that means!"

"I know, Mom is going to spoil Jennifer. That's for sure. She will do things for her that she never did for us."

"Now, don't get jealous, Laura! I will have to give her the attention your father would give her, if he were around today. So, I have to give Jennifer a double dose of love!"

"I can't blame you, Mom. I am sorry, I was just kidding."

"I know that."

Jeanie and Mrs. Secula left at eight o'clock in the evening.

The next day, Laura was started on physiotherapy. Her gait was still wobbly. Her steps were uncertain, and she had difficulty standing up and putting her feet together flat on the floor. For the first two days, she had to use a walker. She was discharged on the fourth day after delivery. The physiotherapist would give her therapy three times a week until she developed a steady gait.

Michael took off the first week Laura was home. He had to do everything for her because she still had an unsteady gait. He did the wash, house cleaning, cooking, and the shopping. He didn't mind it as long as Laura was comfortable. He even prepared snacks for the physiotherapist whenever she came in to exercise Laura's legs.

"Dr. Secula, where did you find your husband? He is so nice and thoughtful and caring."

"Men like him are not born everyday. He was Godsent. I met him in the emergency room at University Hospital. He was the one who took care of my father in the accident ward. Isn't it strange? I lost my father whom I loved and adored, and, through my father's death, I met the kindest and most thoughtful man there is on earth."

"You are really very lucky. Out there it is very hard to find a decent man today. All they are interested in is sex. They are not interested in a relationship."

"I know what you mean. Michael is also a very highly moral man. He had a very good upbringing. He was raised by a priest. He was an orphan. Very early in life, he learned how to give of himself!"

"I wish I would find a husband like him."

"Don't worry, Diane. You will know when the right man comes along. Don't let romance sweep you off your feet. You have to look at the whole person, his character, his principles, and his outlook on life."

Michael shouted from the kitchen, "Diane, your snack is ready whenever you get finished exercising Laura."

"We will be finished in ten minutes, Michael. I can probably join Diane while she is eating her snack."

"What do want to eat?"

"Just ice sherbet, thank you."

Diane helped Laura to the dining table.

"Michael, please join us. You have been doing housework the whole morning. Please take a break."

"I am trying to prepare dinner for us. I want it ready before Mom and Jeanie arrive. Then I will just have to heat it. I will be in shortly, though. Would you care to have a cup of coffee, Laura?"

"No, I will pass. I don't want Jennifer to get constipated. I don't know how much of the coffee will pass through my milk."

"Can I get you lemonade then?"

"That would be fine. Thank you."

As soon as Diane finished her snack, she left. Michael helped Laura back to bed.

"I think I better get you support stockings. You have been on bedrest for so many months now, that I am afraid you might throw an embolus."

"You can look for my maternity support stockings in the closet. I will put them on, if that is what you want."

"Laura, come on. It is what is good for you. I am concerned about you. I worry about your health."

"I am as healthy as can be, only I can't walk straight. I promise you, I will be back to my old self in two more weeks. Then, Diane can stop coming here."

"I know you are very fond of Diane and are worried she will get mugged in the neighborhood."

It was time for Michael to go back to work. Jeanie dropped off Mrs. Secula everyday before she went to work. It was very convenient for her. She worked near Michael and Laura's apartment. Mrs. Secula found a lot of joy in helping Laura take care of Jennifer. She even volunteered to sleep over and take care of Jennifer while Laura rested. She was even willing to come everyday to Michael and Laura's apartment, so that Jennifer did not have to be awakened early in the morning for Michael to take her to Kalina Street.

Three weeks passed. Laura was now on her feet. Mrs. Secula did not have to come everyday, only when Laura needed to go out for groceries or run errands for Michael.

It was Laura's fifth week postpartum. She went to her obstetrician for a check-up. She wanted to go back to work at exactly six weeks postpartum. Even though her co-residents had visited her in the hospital and had sent her flowers after she delivered, she was sure that, deep down, there was that repressed feeling of resentment towards her.

CHAPTER XXVI

Laura had her last postpartum check up May 23, 1985. She also went to Northend Hospital to check her working schedule. She would be on call on the first day she came back to work.

Mrs. Secula was going to take care of Jennifer as planned and agreed upon by Mrs. Secula, Michael, and Laura.

Michael had only one month left for his fellowship. Then he would be an assistant instructor in surgery. He was going to be involved with research work, too. The more scientific papers a doctor wrote, the better the chance of him getting promoted faster in a university setting.

He started working in anatomic pathology in order to brush up on the minutest muscles, vessels, and nerves in the body. He had already signed a one-year contract as an assistant instructor in surgery. He would be scrubbing with residents and would teach anatomical dissection in the medical school. Michael was really looking forward to a few years of academic life while waiting for Laura to finish her surgical residency. Then, they would decide where they would relocate and practice. They both decided that they would choose an area which was conducive for family life.

On June 3rd, 1985, on the busy and bustling surgical floor of the university hospital, an operator could be heard, "Michael Olsire, extension 8119, Dr. Michael Olsire, extension 8119."

Michael answered the telephone page.

"Michael, this is Dr. Daniel Tearcell, I would like to talk to you in my office before you go home today. I want to discuss something with you."

"What is this all about, Dr. Tearcell?"

"I have to talk to you in private. It is something I should not discuss with anyone on the phone; that would be too impersonal."

"I will be there this afternoon after I finish my post-operative rounds. I promised the residents that I would meet them after my last case. Is 4:30 p.m. alright with you, Dr. Tearcell?"

"That would be fine, Michael. I will be waiting for you in my office."

At 3:30 p.m., Michael was making surgical rounds with the residents. They discussed their morbidity and mortality cases. One case that was discussed was a 53-year-old woman with perforated diverticulosis causing fecal excretions into the vagina. The woman had an emergency colostomy done and would be readmitted several weeks later for revision of colostomy and bowel resection.

Another case was a bowel perforation secondary to laparoscopic tubal ligation. This young lady in her thirties was not yet out of the woods. She had had massive peritonitis when she was admitted. She was on massive antibiotics. Michael asked if anyone of the residents had any questions or suggestions.

"Do you think all these cases were handled and managed correctly by us?"

"Absolutely."

"Tomorrow, we are going to discuss risk management. We are going to have discussions on the trend of medico-legal litigation around the country from Florida to California. I will be seeing you tomorrow at two o'clock after the surgical clinic."

By the time the surgical round was finished, it was already 5:00 p.m. Dr. Daniel Tearcell had already left. He left a note for Michael: "I will see you Wednesday, Michael. Sorry I could not wait for you. I will be off tomorrow, Tuesday."

Michael tossed in bed the whole night. Laura was at work. He wanted to talk to someone, but Mrs. Secula and Jennifer were already asleep. He called Laura, but she was in surgery. He wanted to call Father John, but it was already one o'clock in the morning. He did not want to wake him up. So, he decided to read until he fell asleep.

Michael woke up at 6:20 a.m. Mrs. Secula had already prepared breakfast for him; Jennifer was still asleep. Her sleep pattern had been getting better. She woke up only once at 11:00 p.m. and slept soundly the rest of the night.

"Mom, thank you for preparing breakfast for me. I am embarrassed. I should be preparing breakfast for you and Jennifer."

"Don't be embarrassed, Michael. I am used to waking up early and preparing breakfast for Laura and Jeanie."

The phone rang.

"Michael, it must be Laura on the phone. She probably wants to find out how Jennifer made out without her being home."

"I will pick it up, Mom."

"Michael, how are you? How did Mom and Jennifer make out last night? I hope Jennifer did not keep Mom awake all night."

"Well, Laura, you should be proud of our little princess. She went to sleep at nine o'clock, woke up at eleven o'clock, and slept all night afterwards."

"Oh, I can't believe this!"

"But that's how well she behaved last night!"

"Michael, I won't be home tonight. One of the second year residents had an emergency appendectomy. I am supposed to cover for him tonight. We are trying to work out the schedule until he comes back."

"Does that mean four weeks?"

"I don't know yet. I will see you Wednesday night. Please, put Mom on the phone."

Michael handed the phone to Mrs. Secula.

"Mom, I am sorry. I will not be able to come home tonight. I have to cover for another surgical resident. Michael will tell you all about it. I am sorry to impose on you. I hope you understand."

"Laura, stop apologizing. Who else would take care of Jennifer, except her only grandmom who adores her."

"Thank you, Mom."

Later that morning, as soon as Michael had finished scrubbing with the residents, he went to lunch early so he could prepare the risk management lecture he was going to give to the residents.

By two o'clock in the afternoon, all the surgical residents had gathered in the lecture room. Michael stated that, to be a better physician, a doctor should not only take good care of his patients. He should also be well-informed of the laws of the state where he lived and practiced with their application in medico-legal malpractice cases. He should also take risk management courses. For example, in Pennsylvania, error in judgement was not medical malpractice, but the plaintiff lawyer could still get the doctor for failure to diagnose.

"In some sates, the plaintiff lawyers can attach all your assets even before the trial of a case if your insurance coverage is less than the anticipated judgement, especially in a blatant case of medical negligence or medical malpractice. In Pennsylvania, the plaintiff lawyer has to prove that there was fraud on the part of the physician before he can attach a physician's assets, even if there was blatant negligence or blatant malpractice."

"How can a plaintiff lawyer get you for fraud?"

"This is prevalent in some states. Most doctors don't believe in giving informed consent. In California, fraud is being successfully used against obstetricians and, in due time, this will spread all over the country. Just wait until the FDA puts on the labels of birth control pills that the risks in taking birth control pills are stroke, breast cancer, and hypertension. The plaintiff lawyers will have a field day! Unethical plaintiff lawyers have a way of twisting, stretching, and inventing the truth, too. You should not be scared when they include punitive damage. This is one of their ploys to make you settle or scare you into settling a case. Just remember, anyone can sue you. Just because you got sued does not mean you are incompetent or negligent. There are such things as poor results in spite of trying your best. Sometimes, the disease follows its natural course of disaster. But, just as physicians are accountable for their actions, so are patients, lawyers, employers, and healthcare and medical liability insurance companies for trying to set a trend of medical practice."

"Shouldn't unethical plaintiff lawyers be made accountable for filing frivolous suits?"

"Yes, you can countersue them after you win a medical malpractice suit filed frivolously. It is also a myth that lawyers don't sue other lawyers for abuse of the legal process. There is a trend going on in the country. Doctors are fighting back. They are starting to countersue lawyers who file frivolous suits, and they are winning. Also, a few medical societies are even funding the countersuits of the frivolous suits won by defendant physicians. So, this is not a lost cause. Even a defense lawyer can be sued for legal malpractice by a defendant physician if he feels the lawyer screwed up the defense of a malpractice case because of poor preparation or because of a misplaced loyalty to the insurance company rather than to his client, the defendant physician. The insurance company can also be sued for conspiracy, along with the defense lawyer whose loyalty was to the insurance company. Just like any other insurance company, medical liability insurance companies are no different. They exist to make profit. They can do this shrewdly without even arousing the suspicion of naive, insured physicians by contracting with mediocre defense law firms at a lower fee which would not be acceptable to a reputable defense firm. Moreover, this mediocre defense law firm may be taking orders from the medical liability insurance company to talk a client into settling a case in order to keep its contract with the medical liability insurance company. Are these medical liability insurance companies the HMO's of the legal profession? If liability insurance companies decide to go the HMO route in defending their physician clients, they just might find themselves in a morass of litigation by unhappy, harried physicians who feel that their lawsuits have not been defended vigorously by a reputable lawyer. The writing is on the wall! This situation will present itself as soon as the National Data Bank for physicians is in full operation. Reputable legal firms would never go along with manipulation by the medical liability insurance companies. They defend their physician clients vigorously without thought of monetary gain. Reputable legal firms take their legal oath as seriously as reputable doctors do the Hippocratic Oath."

"How do you prevent medical malpractice suits?"

"By developing a relationship with the patient, being honest, and giving informed consent. The country is craving the type of doctor who made house calls, empathized with the patient's emotional distress, and was friendly with the family, in short, a family friend. Patients resent greedy doctors. It does not mean, though, that you will not get sued if you show patients you care and even go out of your way to help them with their problems. Greed is a very powerful emotion and vice; it is like a cancer. Once greed enters into the human mind, the relationship goes out of the window. You must remember that human nature is fickle and unpredictable. You can never predict which patient will turn against you. My only advice is to keep your integrity and dignity intact. Practice good medicine and practice with your conscience. Don't do anything that would be in conflict with your principles and medical judgement. Always practice medicine according to the Hippocratic Oath. You will never go wrong. It might not be financially rewarding, but, on the other hand, you have to live with yourself. Peace of mind is more important than having a lot of money. The patient will perceive it, if you are practicing like a businessman. They will treat you like a businessman."

"What about contingency fees?"

"They are legal in this country. They are illegal in Europe and Japan. The lawyers in this country think this is the only way that justice will be rendered and that the legal system will be accessible to medically injured patients."

"Doesn't it increase healthcare cost?"

"Tremendously, in the form of defensive medicine and overuse of technology."

"What can we do about it?"

"Nothing. Unless the politicians realize this problem, there is nothing we can do but hang on."

"Do you think the government will do something soon?"

"No. Two-thirds of Congress are lawyers. Do you think they will legislate against themselves?"

"You are right."

"What we need are accountability and reevaluation of our moral values."

"I hope it will eventually get to that point."

"Unfortunately, suing doctors frivolously is the easiest way to make tax-free money," said Michael.

"Do doctors being sued go through emotional turmoil like the Post-Stress Syndrome of Vietnam vets?"

"Definitely, I went through that myself. Right now, Dr. Simmons, James Dillon, John Miller, and I are being sued by a lawyer named Robert Smith for inflicting hepatitis and AIDS on Charlie Singleton."

"How appalling!"

"It is true."

"I can't imagine how this family can even think of suing you. You went out of your way to help them all the time while he was in the hospital."

"I was shocked myself. I did not realize you could get sued for caring too much. We do not know how the color of money influences people's minds and thinking. Time will tell why Mrs. Singleton is suing."

"Right now the quality of healthcare is deteriorating and healthcare cost is rising. Expect to see an avalanche of medical malpractice suits to follow in a year or two."

"Why do you say that, Dr. Olsire?"

"The healthcare laws that have been passed by Congress are flawed."

"Which ones?"

"The DRG, the HMO Federal Act of 1973, and the mandatory drug substitution laws. These laws practically make a doctor commit medical malpractice unless he stands up for his patients and educates their families."

"I think doctors should do something about it, like organizing together before it's too late."

"Doctors are a different breed of animal. They are rugged individualists, very independent, and, unless their pocketbook is affected, they will not care. There is so much apathy in the medical profession that, unless all physicians get together and reverse the tide moving against all of us, the healthcare in this country will deteriorate further, and lives will be jeopardized. In the meantime, shrewd healthcare entrepreneurs will be laughing all the way to the bank with their shareholders. More doctors will be accountable for the deteriorating quality of care, and more and more medical malpractice suits will be filed against physicians."

"Will no-fault insurance work for medical malpractice?"

"No, there was a study done in the seventies in one of the western states that, if all the patients who had been injured or damaged by doctors were compensated, the whole healthcare system of that state would be bankrupt. That includes physicians, too."

"Is it true that the medical profession in one year kills more people due to medical malpractice than the Vietnam and Korean Wars did combined?"

"Unfortunately, it is true. The medical profession is not policing itself adequately. There are impaired physicians who are practicing when they should not be. I think the medical profession owes it to the public to stop these impaired physicians from practicing until they are rehabilitated. Organized medicine should think of the public welfare first. It is actually an act of love, not one of punishment, to stop impaired physicians from practicing. But, if the credential committee in a hospital tries to censure an impaired or incompetent physician, the unethical and greedy lawyers who file frivolous medical malpractice suits will be the same lawyers who will defend this type of doctor. It would not be long before a crafty lawyer could figure out how the whole medical staff of a hospital could be sued for letting an incompetent physician continue to practice."

"So what can we do?"

"Nothing. Doctors are all lumped in one basket. Whether you are good or bad, the public perceives you as they perceive bad doctors."

"Isn't that terrible?"

"It is, but there is nothing we can do about it unless we earn back whatever trust the public had in doctors in the past. The physician's image changed dramatically when doctors started advertising! The same thing happened to the image of lawyers. We have to show the public that we are humane by giving more free care to the poor and uninsured. We have to encourage voluntaryism among physicians."

"How do we conduct ourselves then?"

"Well, just be yourself. Do unto the patient whatever you would have done unto any member of your family or yourself. DO NO HARM!"

"Do you think socialized medicine will be adopted here?"

"No, the lawyers and insurance industry will vigorously fight it. Insurance companies would be abolished. Litigation would be curtailed. In Canada, England, and other European countries, medical malpractice suits are screened before they are even filed in court. There are no expensive depositions unless the court puts out a decree. As I have said before, there is no contingency fee allowed, and lawyers who file frivolous suits are sanctioned. In Japan, lawyers are looked down upon. There are only 10,000 lawyers in the whole country. In Pennsylvania alone, there are almost 35,000 lawyers, and Philadelphia has 14,000 of them. Moreover, the unethical, greedy lawyers in Philadelphia try to work medical malpractice lawsuits backwards. They file the frivolous lawsuits first. Then, if they can't find an expert to testify against the doctor, they try to intimidate the physician in order to extort money from him. Sometimes they use the name of an unqualified physician who is supposed to be an expert witness. They even try to settle a case by asking the physician to sign that he will not countersue them later. The defendant physician has one recourse; he can refuse to be deposed unless the plaintiff lawyer can produce a qualified expert witness. Those stupid lawyers who file stupid, frivolous suits should be punished because they are increasing healthcare cost and clogging the already overloaded judicial system. In Pennsylvania, if a frivolous suit is dropped according to Rule 229, the unethical lawyer can be countersued. Hopefully, lawyers will soon have tremors when

Rule 11 becomes applicable not only in federal courts but in state courts; abuse of the legal process will decrease tremendously because of the fines and sanctions against unethical lawyers."

"I could not agree more."

Michael continued, "I think what we need are more aggressive defense lawyers. I think we need more M.D. J.D.'s. But most M.D.'s end up as plaintiff lawyers."

"What has litigation done to specialty medicine?"

"Obstetrics is really under fire. More and more obstetricians have quit delivering babies. Some states are even paying the medical liability insurance of obstetricians so that they will deliver Medicaid patients."

"Do you feel that, since there is so much stress, it might not even be worth it to be a doctor?"

"It depends on your priorities in life. Some of the obstetricians increase their own liability risks, too, in the way they practice."

"In what way?"

"By using too much technology in their offices. For example, having an Ultrasound in your office to increase your revenue. If a physician misses a diagnosis by using his own ultrasound, or if the capability is not comparable with the one being used in a level II ultrasound center, the plaintiff lawyer can hang him for that. Billing patients for pap smears is another bad idea. A doctor becomes an agent of the laboratory when he bills for the pap smear. If the laboratory makes a mistake in the pap smear, the physician is as liable as the laboratory. Drawing blood in the office and sending it to the laboratory isn't wise either. The physician is as liable as the laboratory, if the specimen is lost or if the blood values of tests are inaccurate because of poor quality control. The problem here is that the doctor makes a five-dollar fee for every patient whose blood is drawn, and he can also make profit by charging more to the patient or to the patient's insurance company. When a plaintiff lawyer portrays the physician as a greedy entrepreneur, he will really have his day in court. Also unethical is referring patients to imaging centers where the physician is a stockholder. This is a clear conflict of interest. The patient should be told about it and the percentage of stock the physician owns. Referring patients to a medical equipment outfit which the physician owns is unethical as well. This is another clear conflict of interest. The patient should be told about it. There are laws in each state specifying the percentage of interest the physician may own and that the patient should be told about it.

"An obstetrician must get informed consent when he is giving the epidural anaesthesia himself. He should inform the patient that sudden hypotension may decrease the amount of oxygen available to the fetus and that this may compromise the baby neurologically later on in life. The thin-walled epidural veins may also be inadvertently punctured during placement of the epidural catheter. A high level of anaesthetic drug may go to the fetus. Epidural anaesthesia may prolong labor, thereby increasing the rate of pitocin induction which in turn increases operative and sometimes traumatic vaginal deliveries and the Caesarean section rate. In Ireland, the Caesarean section rate is only 3%. Epidural anaesthesia is not used in that country. There are also very few lawyers there.

"The use of vacuum extractor is not a new phenomenon, but the mother should be told that tentorial tears are a possibility. Risks of vaginal lacerations and extension of episiotomies should be explained to the patient before the vacuum extractor is used. The plaintiff lawyers will always find a way of calling all these obstetrical instruments destructive if injury to the baby or mother occurs.

"The specialty medicine colleges put out guidelines that have to be followed by practitioners in each specialty. For example, with obstetricians, if the guidelines put out by the college are not followed, and the baby or mother is injured, the plaintiff lawyer may use the guideline to bolster his case."

"It must be so overwhelming to practice obstetrics."

"It is very stressful. If things go wrong, two lives are immediately jeopardized."

"Now I know why obstetricians are leaving obstetrics."

"You can't blame them."

"In Pennsylvania, the statute of limitation for an injured baby is 21 years, whereas in other states, like California, it is only eight years.

"Another area of litigation that you should be aware of pertains to therapeutic risks. No matter what kind of drug you've prescribed, there are always risks of untoward reactions. Be sure you tell the patient about it.

"In blood transfusion litigation, always have an informed consent concerning the risk of hepatitis and AIDS. This is what Robert Smith is trying to get us on. It does not matter whether it's an emergency or not, you still must tell the patient."

"This is the most interesting conference we've ever had."

"We should do it more often."

"I am glad you enjoyed it," Michael said, "You are at least informed about the litigation going on around the country."

"Thank you, Michael."

"You are all welcome. I have to go. I will see you tomorrow."

CHAPTER XXVII

Michael went directly to the office of Dr. Daniel Tearcell. He was busy reading when Michael walked into his office.

"Michael, make yourself comfortable. Do you want anything to drink?"

"No, thank you, Dr. Tearcell."

Michael seated himself across from Dr. Tearcell. He noticed that Dr. Tearcell was deep in thought. Michael broke the silence.

"Dr. Tearcell, I am sure you did not ask me here to discuss something trivial. I presume from your facial expressions that you are vacillating on whether or not to tell me something."

"Michael, I don't know how to start. I lay awake last night, thinking how I would tell someone who is so devoted to his work this bad news."

"Dr. Tearcell, do you mean to say that my HIV and Western blot tests are both positive?"

Dr. Tearcell, in a sad, choked voice, said, "I am very sorry, Michael, to break this bad news to you. I wish I could say something different, but you have to know."

"Oh, my God! I hope Laura and Jennifer did not get it from me. I would never be able to forgive myself if they did!"

Michael put his hands over his face and started sobbing.

"My worst fears have been confirmed. I have been feeling very tired for the past three months. I did not tell Laura; I did not want to worry her in her condition."

"Do you think you could have infected Laura?"

"I am not sure. My HIV and Western blot tests were both negative one month after we found out Laura was pregnant. We stopped making love during her fourth month because of her irritable uterus which resulted from her fibroid."

"Laura will have to have HIV and Western blot tests done in order to find out if she has it or not. It is better that she get it done here. I will keep everything confidential. But you have to tell the chief of surgery, Michael."

Michael, still sobbing, responded, "I want to tell my wife first before I tell anyone else. I have to call her at the hospital now to see if she can talk her mom into taking our baby with her tonight. We need time together to discuss this problem."

Michael dialed Northend Hospital and had Laura paged. Laura was busy changing a patient's surgical dressing, and the nurse wanted to take the message. Michael insisted that he would hold on and wait for Laura to finish whatever she was doing.

"Michael, what's going on? Your message sounded so urgent. Is something wrong?"

"Laura, please ask Mom if she can take Jennifer home with her tonight. We need to talk."

"Did some catastrophe happen at your hospital?"

"No, it is about my career. I will tell you all about it when I see you tonight. Call me at the hospital as soon as you get home. I do not want Mom to see me in this condition. I don't want to upset her."

"I will call you as soon as Jeanie picks them up."

"Laura, don't bother preparing dinner. I will just eat in the cafeteria."

"Whatever you say, Michael."

"Goodbye."

Laura was puzzled, "Why does Michael sound so sad?"

Laura went home hurriedly as soon as she finished her post-operative rounds. She raced along the expressway. Jeanie was already at their apartment to pick up Mrs. Secula.

"Mom, do you think you can take Jennifer home with you tonight?"

"Laura, I would gladly take Jennifer with me not only tonight, but for the rest of her growing years."

Laura hugged Mrs. Secula.

"Mom, I know I can always depend on you and Jeanie."

Laura hugged Jeanie, too.

"We are a family, Laura. We have to hang on together."

Michael did not arrive until about 7:00 p.m.

"Michael, you look so sad and washed out."

His shoulders were drooping, too. His eyes were bloodshot from crying. Laura started crying. She hugged and kissed him.

"Michael, please talk to me. What is going on?"

"Laura, I don't even know how I will start. Everything is so blurred and grim. My life and career are both hanging in the balance."

Laura wiped her tears. "Michael, let's sit down and talk. We can't let our emotions rule our minds. We have to think and talk intelligently."

"Laura, my HIV and Western blot tests are both positive. Dr. Tearcell told me the news today. He tried to talk to me Monday, but I missed my appointment with him. Tuesday, he was off. Since Monday, I have been tossing in bed. I called you at the hospital Monday and Tuesday nights, but both times you were in surgery. I felt so alone. I could not tell anyone about my fears of the tests being positive. For the past two nights, I have not been sleeping. So, when Dr. Tearcell talked to me today in his office, that was just the last straw. I could not control myself. I started crying like a small boy. I could not believe what I heard. Dr. Tearcell was very upset that he had to tell me the bad news."

"Michael, crying does not make you a lesser man. It makes you more human."

"Thank you, Laura. I don't know how to tell you without upsetting you that you have to have HIV and Western blot tests, too. You have to have it done at my hospital. Dr. Tearcell promised me that everything will be confidential."

"Michael, I don't think you have infected me. I will get it done to be sure and also to protect Jennifer."

"God forbid that both of us would have it! Who would take care of Jennifer?"

"Michael, we will cross that bridge when we get there. I want you to know that my love for you has not diminished and will not diminish because of your affliction with AIDS. We are in this together. We are going to put to better use whatever time together God has intended for us. You can always count on me, Michael. We will always be together for better or for worse. Are you going to tell Father John and all our friends?"

"I have to wait until I talk to the chief of surgery. I have to meet him tomorrow morning at 8:00 a.m. I am expecting the worst."

"Michael, please think positive. When are we going to tell Mom and Jeanie?"

"As soon as I have talked to my chief."

"That means we can tell them tomorrow night."

"I think so."

"Michael, I can assure you that Mom and Jeanie will be very supportive of us. They will understand our situation."

"I hope so."

Michael and Laura tossed in bed. Both of them could not sleep.

Michael grasped Laura's hand and said, "You know what this means."

"I know that we will not be able to make love anymore, but that is not the only way to show affection to a loved one. Being thoughtful is another way. Cuddling and touching will be more than enough. The most important thing is that we have each other and that we communicate very well. We just have to hope for the best."

"Laura, I don't know what I would have done if I hadn't had you and Jennifer in my life. You and Jennifer are my inspiration. I want to live longer. I want to see Jennifer grow up."

"So do I. Let's get some sleep, Michael. I am going to have Jeanie and Mom stay for dinner tomorrow. We will have to tell Father John tomorrow as well. You have to call John Miller and James Dillon, too. They both took care of Charlie. How about Tom Wittle?"

"I should probably tell him, too."

Michael and Laura woke up early. They both had a cup of coffee. Laura kissed Michael before she left, "Keep your chin up, Michael. It is not the end of the world. We will survive."

"I hope so."

Laura was preoccupied with Michael's illness while she was driving. She did not even realize that she had passed through a red light. A female cop stopped her.

"What is the matter with you, lady? Don't you realize that you just passed through a red light? You could have killed someone or could have had a head-on-collision with a tractor truck."

Laura did not utter a word. She just looked at the cop with her sad, tear-filled blue eyes and nodded.

The female cop bent over to look at her closely. "What is the matter with you? Are you in pain? Is something wrong with you? You look as if the problems of the whole world have just fallen on your shoulders. I will let you go this time, but be careful the rest of your way. I don't want you to have an accident and become a statistic."

Laura replied tersely, "Thank you," and continued driving.

In the meantime, Michael was waiting for Dr. Ebstein in his office. Dr. Ebstein finally arrived at 8:15 a.m.. Michael noticed that he looked stern and formal.

"Michael, what can I do for you today?"

"I have to tell you something very serious. I was just told I had positive HIV and Western blot tests. That means I have AIDS."

"Where do you think you got it from?"

"From operating on a patient, Charlie Singleton. He expired in December, 1983."

"Where do you think he got it from?"

"He was a drug abuser. Several other homeless people from his group have been diagnosed with AIDS as well and have been admitted to this hospital."

"What do you think you should do?"

"I don't know, Dr. Ebstein."

"Well, as far as I am concerned, you are terminated. I can't have you scrubbing in the operating room. I would be exposing patients and residents unnecessarily to AIDS."

"But, Dr. Ebstein, I still have one month with my fellowship! I have already signed my contract as an assistant instructor for next year!"

"Michael, you have outlived your usefulness. How can I let you scrub when you have AIDS? This will not be fair to all the people working in the operating room."

"I understand that, Dr. Ebstein, but I can do research work."

"That's out of the question. There is no vacancy in the research department."

"So, what options do I have then?"

"Nothing, but to quit!"

"Dr. Ebstein, where is your compassion? You are actually cutting my life away. Where are the caring and compassion that the medical profession preaches? From you, of all people, I least expected to hear this. You have not even uttered one kind word to a colleague who is really down. Instead of showing me a ray of hope, you have shown me nothing but arrogance and callousness. Where is your heart? You don't deserve to replace Dr. Simmons. You do not even qualify to shine his shoes. As far as I am concerned, you are a typical medical bureaucrat. You are all for yourself. You don't even care that I will not have healthcare insurance coverage, even though you are well aware that I have developed a preexisting condition. How can you behave like this? Please look at yourself in front of a mirror so you can see your own mask."

"Enough, Michael. This conversation has to end before I lose my temper and throw you out of my office. You can pack your bags."

Michael went home hurriedly. Mrs. Secula and Jeanie were already there preparing the dining table. As soon as Michael walked in, Mrs. Secula knew something was wrong. Michael's hair was disheveled; he looked so haggard and exhausted. There was so much sadness in those big, blue eyes. Mrs. Secula took Michael aside and asked, "Michael, is there something wrong?"

"Mom, a lot of things are going wrong in our lives. I have just been diagnosed as having AIDS. A while ago, Dr. Ebstein terminated my contract. Now, when I really need it, I will not have insurance coverage because of what I have. Laura's insurance will not cover me either because it is another commercial insurance company. I wish the University would let me pay for my insurance coverage through them."

Jeanie, who had overheard, came over and said, "Michael, Mom and I will always look out for you, Laura, and Jennifer. I know it must have been heartbreaking to hear the bad news. Nothing is changed. Mom and I love you just the same. It does not make you a lesser person just because you have AIDS. We will always be there for you and Laura and Jennifer."

"Let us have something to eat. Then Michael can call Father John. I don't know how he will take this. I hope nothing happens to him."

After dinner, Michael decided to drink a glass of wine. He was quite jittery. He was pacing the floor.

"Laura, do you want to talk to Father John first? I don't know how I will get started."

"Michael, please try to compose yourself. Father John should be able to handle this pretty well. Please do not underestimate him."

Michael dialed the number and got Father John right away.

"Father John, this is Michael. When can you come for Jennifer's christening?"

"Anytime after this weekend."

"How about next weekend?"

"That would be fine. I will take the flight at 8:00 p.m., and you can pick me up at the airport."

"We will see you then, Father John. Do you want to talk to Laura, Father John?"

"I would love to."

"Father John, we will be expecting you then. Jennifer is getting bigger and heavier everyday. I am sure you are eager to hold her."

"Absolutely."

Laura hung up the phone and looked at Michael. Michael explained, "I did not have the heart to tell Father John the bad news. I will tell him after Jennifer's christening."

"That's fine with me, Michael. I think you ought to call Dr. Simmons and Debbie later before they find out from Dr. Ebstein."

"I will call him later."

Mrs. Secula and Jeanie left at 9:00 p.m.. They both looked as sad as Michael and Laura.

Michael called Dr. Simmons.

"How are you, Michael? What is up?"

"Dr. Simmons, I don't know how to start. Have you talked to Dr. Ebstein?"

"No. Why would I talk to him? I can't even stand that arrogant and callous man. It was an insult to me that the University decided to replace me with that type of medical bureaucrat."

"Well, he just terminated me today after I told him that my HIV and Western blot tests were both positive. I offered to work as a researcher, but he refused to hear of it. I will be losing my healthcare insurance benefit at the time I need it most."

"How can that heartless man do this to you? He must be taking out on you the fact that you are one of my favorite residents. He is trying to get back at me through you. I will talk to the board of trustees about your healthcare benefits. Don't worry, Michael, I will look after you and Laura. If you need help, call me or Debbie. I will call you back tomorrow after I talk to the board of trustees. How is Laura taking it?"

"She is taking it better than me."

"May I talk to Laura, please?"

"Hold on, Dr. Simmons."

Laura took the phone from Michael.

"Laura, how are you holding up? I am sorry to hear about Michael's illness. You can always count on me and Debbie. Please do not hesitate to call us."

"Thank you, Dr. Simmons. Knowing that we have friends who genuinely care about us makes our load lighter. Please tell Debbie I said hello."

"I will, and hang in there. We love both of you. Do you mind if I tell Jorge and Estela? They are both very fond of you and Michael."

"You should also tell James Dillon, John Miller, and Tom Wittle. They all took care of Charlie Singleton."

"I will call them up then. Good night, Laura."

"Thank you, Dr. Simmons."

"You are welcome, Laura."

"Remember, Jennifer will be baptized next Sunday. Do you think that you and Debbie can come for lunch at my mother's house?"

"Debbie and I will drop by. Thank you for inviting us. Goodbye, Laura."

"'We will see you then."

The next morning, Dr. Simmons went to the University to discuss the healthcare benefits of Michael with the chief of the Board of Trustees.

"How are you, Dr. Simmons? What a pleasant surprise! We thought you had forgotten us since your retirement."

"How can I forget the University where I taught for forty years? How can I forget the University which preached caring and compassion to its medical students and residents all these years, but yet in one unusual case treats one of its alumni arrogantly and compassionlessly?"

"Why are you so upset, Jay?"

"Well, Dr. Ebstein abruptly terminated Dr. Michael Olsire yesterday after he found out from him that both his HIV and Western blot tests were positive. He did not show one bit of compassion. The young man is scared enough for his life, his wife, and his daughter. This is not the way to treat someone who is already down on his luck. It's like stabbing him in the face and in the back.

"Mr. Armstrong, please find it in your heart to cover the healthcare insurance of Michael according to his contract for the start of the new fiscal year. It is not going to drain your budget."

"I know, Dr. Simmons, but we can't allow him to work in the operating room or else we will be exposing the medical students and patients to AIDS."

"AIDS is transferred sexually or by contact of broken skin with body fluids. That is how Michael became infected with Charlie Singleton's blood. You can at least give him a job in a research department."

"But we have no opening."

"Is that what Dr. Ebstein told you?"

"No, our quota has been filled."

"You can put him in an area in which he would not have to deal with patients or the public."

"We can't take that chance. We will cover his insurance for the rest of the contract that was agreed upon for one year. After that, he will be on his own."

"Thank you, Mr. Armstrong. I will tell Michael. You know what? You better get yourself a lawyer to find out your responsibility to any resident stricken with AIDS. Otherwise, you will be finding yourself in court."

"Are you trying to say that you will talk Michael Olsire into suing us?"

"Only if you don't keep your promise to cover his healthcare benefits and disability insurance. Not only will I spend the money for Michael to sue University Hospital, but I will also cut off the donations to the University which I give every year. I will also dismantle the trust fund I set up for the University. I hope I have made myself clear. This is not a threat; it is a promise. Good day, Mr. Armstrong."

Mr. Armstrong could not believe that Dr. Jay Simmons had said such harsh words to him. Everyone else at University Hospital knew not to mess around with Dr. Simmons' circle of favorite surgical residents and fellows. He could really let go with his Irish temper otherwise.

Mr. Armstrong immediately telephoned Dr. Ebstein and told him about the conversation he'd just had.

"Dr. Ebstein, Dr. Simmons was here, and he was really fuming. I thought he was going to strangulate me with his bare hands. We will have to continue the healthcare benefits of Michael Olsire for another year; otherwise, we will be in a lot of trouble."

"Are you going to yield to this blackmail gimmick of Jay Simmons?"

"You don't know how powerful this man is! He has accumulated wealth from investing his royalties from writing medical textbooks. It would be a big financial drain to the hospital if he carried out his threat. It will be cheaper for the hospital to continue the healthcare benefits of Michael Olsire rather than making Jay Simmons mad."

"Well, we have to play his game then. We will continue paying for Michael Olsire's healthcare benefits and disability insurance for one year according to his contract."

"I think this is the best decision that we can make."

Dr. Jay Simmons called Michael.

"Michael, everything is taken care of. You will continue to be covered by the hospital healthcare benefits, and your disability insurance will be in force after ninety days. I would like to drop by so I can discuss your treatment with you. I know a very good infectious disease man in the city. Do you mind if I drop by your apartment now?"

"I would love to see you, Dr. Simmons. To me you are not only my mentor, but also my friend."

"I will be there in thirty minutes. I will just get breakfast from the cafeteria. Do you want me to get something for you in the cafeteria?"

"No, thank you, Dr. Simmons. Laura cooked me some hot breakfast before she went to work. Jennifer is staying with my mother-in-law until we hear about Laura's HIV test in a week."

"Michael, what can I say? You and Laura have so much on your minds. I am glad that you are both strong and committed to each other. You are both under a lot of pressure. I hope that just by talking to you and Laura, I am able to help you one way or another. I will see you in a few minutes."

Michael was pacing the living room floor of their apartment when Dr. Simmons knocked at the door.

Michael shook the hand of Dr. Simmons. Dr. Simmons gave Michael a pat on his shoulder.

"Michael, let us sit down and talk. I took the liberty of calling Dr. McIntyre today. He is going to see us this afternoon. I am going to go with you to his office. I hope you don't mind my interference. I just want to free Laura from the worry of taking you back and forth to the doctor."

"Dr. Simmons, it is very thoughtful of you to think and care about us the way you do. I don't know whether we will be able to repay you in the future."

"I talked to Mr. Armstrong today about a research position for you. He told me that their quota had been filled two months ago. I asked him to find a position for you that would not require patient contact."

"Thank you, Dr. Simmons."

By twelve noon, Dr. Simmons and Michael had reminisced about their days at University Hospital.

"Michael, have you heard from your gang yet?"

"Not yet, Dr. Simmons. I guess everyone is as shocked as I am."

"I can imagine. I hope John Miller is not taking it very hard. After he dropped the knife on your hand and you bled during surgery, he was quite depressed for six months. I had to send him to a psychiatrist. I hope he isn't taking this news too poorly."

"I hope so, too."

"Well, let us go. It is hard to find a parking spot in Center City around this time. I don't want us to be late. Dr. McIntyre just squeezed us in the last slot."

Dr. McIntyre was a kindly man of around fifty. When he saw Dr. Simmons and Michael, he gave them both a very firm handshake. His handshake was so tight that Michael thought he was trying to hold on to him.

"Dr. Simmons, Dr. Olsire, please follow me to my consultation rom. I wanted to see you as my last patient so I could talk to you longer. Michael, I am sorry to hear that you got afflicted with this disease. I hope the medical establishment does something about the plight of residents and fellows in training when they get infected with AIDS while taking care of patients. The way hospital administrators treat healthcare workers with AIDS is a major disgrace. They are usually left with a ruined career without any healthcare benefits."

"I can't agree with you more. I would have had the same problem had it not been for the intervention of Dr. Simmons. My healthcare coverage was about to be terminated by Dr. Ebstein. I am glad Dr. Simmons cared enough for me to go to the university and talk to the chairman of the board."

"Michael, I will have to do a complete physical examination on you in the examining room."

"I will go out to the waiting room and read some magazines and newspapers."

"We will call you as soon as I am finished examining Michael, Dr. Simmons." Dr. Simmons left.

"Dr. McIntyre, I am worried about my wife. In your experience, does it take four months for the HIV test to become positive after an initial negative HIV test?"

"Michael, it is very hard to answer your question. Did your wife get tested, too, after you found out about your positive test results?"

"Yes, Dr. Daniel Tearcell did it. He is supposed to call me in two days."

"Well, in that case, call me after you get the test result of your wife."

"I will do that."

"Michael, your lungs are clear. Have you lost weight?"

"Just a couple of pounds. I have not been eating well since I received the bad news."

"How about diarrhea? Fever? Sweats?"

"Nothing like that. I am just tired."

"How about chronic cough?"

"None."

"Do you smoke?"

"No."

"I want to take a chest X-Ray on you. I want to start you on AZT. This is a very expensive drug. It costs about $10,000 for a one-year treatment. I will call the company who makes it to see if they will give it to you at cost since you are a physician.

"Call me tomorrow; I should have an answer for you. I can give you some capsules here. Before you take them, I want to see how the level of your T-cells are."

"Thank you for giving me the AZT. I will go to the university hospital and have the T-cell count tomorrow. I should have the result for you within seven to ten days."

After examining Michael, Dr. McIntyre pat his back. "We have to see how your T-cells are, and then we will go from there. You do not have full blown AIDS. Let us keep our fingers crossed."

"Thank you, Dr. McIntyre, and thank you for your optimism."

They returned to Dr. Simmons and told him the results.

"Dr. McIntyre, thank you for seeing Michael today. It is very uplifting to know that he does not have a full blown manifestations of AIDS. Thanks again and have a nice day."

"I will call you with the result of the T-cell count as soon as I hear from the university. Thank you, Dr. McIntyre."

Dr. Simmons and Michael went to a restaurant to have a snack.

"Michael, I feel so relieved. I hope AZT will prevent the progress of your disease."

"I hope so, too, Dr. Simmons. Let's just hope for the best. I am going to call Laura as soon as I get home. I am sure she will be happy to hear the good news."

"I am sure she will."

As soon as they finished eating, Dr. Simmons drove Michael back to his apartment. He immediately called Laura. Laura was still in the operating room. He left a message for her to call him at home. Michael fell asleep on the living room sofa.

Ring===Ring===Ring

Michael looked at the clock. It was almost four. He picked up the phone. It was Laura. Her voice was muffled, and she sounded worried. "Michael, what's up?"

"Laura, Dr. Simmons took me to an infectious disease specialist today. He was optimistic. I am going to have my T-cells checked at the university hospital tomorrow. Depending on the number of T-cells, he will put me on AZT to obviate the progress of the disease."

"That's wonderful, Michael. You made my day. I will be coming home soon. We have to call Jorge and Estela, John Miller, and Tom Wittle tonight."

"Do you want me to have dinner ready?"

"No, I already ordered sandwiches for us. I will see you soon."

Laura was exhausted by the time she got home. She was scrubbed in the operating room the whole day. The elderly lady they operated on had ruptured colon secondary to obstruction of a fulminating, extremely malignant, rectosigmoid tumor. The patient had to be transferred to the ICU for close monitoring.

"Michael, I am not sure whether this poor lady will make it. She does not even have relatives to look after her. Her neighbors became suspicious when she did not come out of the house for two days. The cops were called in, and they opened the door for the neighbor. The neighbor found her lying at the foot of the bed."

"That's a shame."

"I know it is. This situation is happening all over the country."

Ring===Ring===Ring

Laura answered the phone, "Hello, may I help you?"

"This is Dr. Tearcell. May I talk to Michael please?"

Laura gave the phone to Michael. "Yes, Dr. Tearcell. How is my wife's test?"

"Michael, I have good news for you. They are both negative. Please tell your wife."

"Thank you, Dr. Tearcell. Laura, your HIV and Western blot are both negative. Thank God for that."

"We have to call Mom and Jeanie."

Laura dialed her mother's number.

"Mom, my AIDS test is negative. Michael was taken to the infectious disease specialist today by Dr. Simmons, and he does not have any symptoms of fullblown AIDS. He will have his T-cells checked, and the doctor will put him on AZT depending on the outcome of the T-cells testing."

"I am glad to hear that, Laura. We will see you Sunday. I will just keep Jennifer here until the christening. When is Father John coming?"

"Saturday. Michael and I will pick him up at the airport."

Laura got off the phone with her mother and then said to Michael, "Michael, let's call Jorge and Estela first."

Michael dialed Estela and Jorge's number, but it was busy.

"Let's try John Miller."

Michael dialed John Miller's number. His wife answered, "John was just called for an emergency surgery in the hospital. I will have him call you as soon as he arrives. How is your little princess?"

"We are going to have her christened this Sunday. Father John is going to do the honors."

"Tell Father John we said hello."

"I will do that. Bye."

"Laura, I lost the number of Dr. Wittle. I will have to call the personnel department tomorrow to see if he left his forwarding address."

Mrs. Secula and Jeanie did all the preparation for Jennifer's christening. They did not want to burden Laura with it. She had been so busy working, moonlighting, and worrying about Michael's illness that she did not have time to worry about food. Jeanie was going to be the godmother. The christening would be after the last Sunday mass.

On June 30th, 1985, Laura and Michael picked up Father John at the airport. Michael was in a pensive mood. He was trying to decide whether he would tell Father John about his illness before the christening or after.

"Father John, do you think you can stay longer with us?"

"I can't, Michael. We are trying to renovate the church plumbing and air conditioning. I am involved in fund-raising. I will have to leave around six tomorrow evening. Why do you ask?"

"Well, Laura and I would like to discuss something very important with you as soon as we finish dinner tonight."

"Alright, after dinner we will talk."

As soon as they reached the apartment, Laura hurriedly reheated the meal she had prepared two nights ago.

"Laura, you have indeed become a good cook. This lasagna really tastes good."

"I am glad you like it, Father John. Would you care for a glass of wine?"

"I would love one, Laura."

After thirty minutes, everyone was finished with dinner. Laura cleared the dining room table and washed the dishes. She was trying to give Michael and Father John the chance to talk alone.

"Father John, I don't really want to break this bad news tonight, but we will have no chance to talk after the christening. Father John, I tested positive for AIDS."

"My God, Michael! How did you get it?"

"From a patient named Charlie Singleton whose wife and children are now suing me, Dr. Simmons, Dr. Dillon, and Dr. Miller."

"What an injustice!"

"It is a long story, Father. I was operating on Charlie Singleton when my assistant, John Miller, accidentally dropped the knife on my hand, and I got cut. It was no one's fault. I had been tested regularly, but it became positive more than two weeks ago. I could not tell you this bad news on the phone when we called about Jennifer's christening. I am sorry I had to tell you tonight."

"Michael, we have to put everything in the hands of God. Everything happens for a purpose. Every misfortune can turn into an opportunity. We cannot question His wisdom, why sometimes He sends each and everyone of us different kinds of misfortunes. We only have to trust Him."

"Thank you, Father John. That is exactly the pep talk I expected from you."

"Laura, why don't you come in and join us? You have been cleaning in the kitchen for a while now."

"I will as soon as I am finished. Would you like to drink more wine or would you rather have coffee?"

"Nothing, thank you. Just sit with us so we can talk."

Laura seated herself between Michael and Father John.

"Laura, I can't thank you enough for all your kindness, concern, and support for my nephew. You are a gem."

"Father John, that's what a committed marriage is all about. You have to take both the good times and the bad. Michael and I have a very stable, solid marriage. Nothing can destroy it."

"That is what I wanted to hear from you, Laura. I know I don't have to worry about Michael. He has a very devoted, loving wife."

On Sunday, July 1st, 1985, Laura, Michael, and Father John woke up early so that they could go to the Secula residence. By 10:00 a.m., Jennifer was just waking up. She started crying when she saw her mom and dad and Father John. Laura took her so she could bathe her after giving her milk. Jennifer was playful while being bathed. She could hardly keep her hands away from the Johnson's Baby Powder. Finally, Laura changed her outfit. Jennifer was going to wear the same christening outfit she had worn.

Everyone already at the house went to the church. The other guests were not expected until after two o'clock. Jeanie invited some of her officemates. Laura and Michael had invited about ten people including Dr. Simmons and Debbie. Mrs. Secula had invited some of her relatives from South Philadelphia.

Jennifer was quite cooperative during the christening ceremony. She was smiling while the baptismal water was being poured on her head. After the ceremony, the guests followed the Seculas and Olsires back to the Secula residence for lunch.

Debbie and Dr. Simmons arrived a little bit late. They had to go to the monastery in their neighborhood to visit the Mother General who was visiting on her way back to Germany. Dr. Simmons stayed behind so they could talk to Laura and Michael.

"Michael, how do you feel?"

"I feel tired, but I do not have the other symptoms of AIDS. I am waiting for the T-cell report to see how much AZT I will have to take. I should be hearing from Dr. McIntyre in a couple of days."

"Please, let me know how you make out."

"I will, Dr. Simmons. Thank you for your interest in my welfare."

"Michael, you and Laura and all the doctors that I have trained are my friends. All of you who conscientiously follow my teachings are Hippocratic medicine's future. I am akin to all of you. It is almost five o'clock. I think we better say goodbye to everyone."

"We can leave together. We will have to drive Father John to the airport."

"We have to say goodbye to Mrs. Secula and Jeanie, too."

Dr. Simmons and his daughter walked over to Mrs. Secula and Jeanie.

"Mrs. Secula, thank you for a lovely party and for inviting me and Debbie. You have to be congratulated. You have raised two lovely girls."

"Thank you, Dr. Simmons. Thank you for your kindness, support and concern for Laura and Michael."

"It is our pleasure."

Debbie and Dr. Simmons left for home. Now, it was Father John's turn to say goodbye. "Mrs. Secula, Jeanie, thank you for your support and for caring about Michael," he said in a choking voice, trying to control his emotions.

"I will try to come back again soon to see you all. Goodbye."

Jennifer was crying when Laura, Michael, and Father John left. Laura ran back to her and kissed her.

"Mom, we will let you know how Michael's T-cells are, and we will then decide if Jennifer can stay with us."

"Laura, don't worry about it. This is more convenient for Jennifer. She does not awaken easily."

"Thanks, Mom," Laura said to Mrs. Secula. Laura ran to the car in the driveway, trying to control her emotions.

The drive to the airport did not take long. The airport was not busy at all. This was one of the slowest days at the airport. Michael found a parking space right away. As soon as they arrived at the ticket counter, the passengers were getting ready to board for South Bend, Indiana. Father John kissed Laura and Michael; he was in a hurry to board the plane. He did not want Laura and Michael to see that he was ready to cry.

As soon as the plane got off the ground, Laura and Michael left the airport.

"Michael, let us go to St. John Neumann's church before we go home."

"Alright, we can make a novena that whatever I have I will be able to deal with well. I have to pray for acceptance. I have to pray for strength and courage and that God will help me bear this disease without my spirit being broken."

"Michael, I think God's greatest gift to you is your faith. I never heard you say 'Why me?' since you have been diagnosed."

"Laura, we have to accept whatever sufferings God sends us. Actually, sufferings are gifts from God. They make us take stock of ourselves and give us an opportunity for emotional and spiritual growth. God is fair. He would never send us crosses which we couldn't handle. I believe in that."

"So do I."

By the time Michael and Laura reached the church, it was already locked. The gift shop was locked, too.

"We will come back on the night I am off. We will just have to say our novena at home."

Michael was opening the apartment door when the phone rang. He quickly picked up the phone. It was John Miller from Ohio.

"Michael, I am heartbroken with the news about you. I have not been sleeping since Dr. Simmons called me two days ago. I am sorry. I wish things were different for you. My carelessness has really ruined your career and your future life with Laura and Jennifer."

"We both agreed after the incident happened that it was an accident. Stop blaming yourself, John. Just pray that I will be able to deal with it emotionally and spiritually without my spirits breaking down. Laura, my best friend and my wife, has given me the most support. She has been a tower of strength in this adversity. I could not have asked God for a better wife."

Laura, overhearing the conversation, said, "My God, I just have to replay what I have heard just now every time you get upset with me!"

"Hold on, John."

Michael turned to his wife. "Laura, I meant what I said."

"I am just kidding, Michael."

On the other end, John said, "Let me talk to Laura, Michael."

Michael handed the phone to Laura. "Laura, I am sorry for everything. If there is anything I can do for both of you, please feel free to call us. My wife wants to talk to you."

Mrs. Miller got on the phone. "Laura, I am very sorry to hear about Michael. Rest assured that John and I are both praying for you."

"Thank you, Ann. The shock is over. We are dealing with the reality now. Michael and I will make it because we really love each other, and we have a relationship. Our love for each other is based on spiritual and intellectual grounds. I wish things were different; the years that God will grant him will be the best years of our lives together. We are very lucky. All of our friends have been good to us. We could not have asked for better friends."

Laura and Ann could not control their emotions now. They both started crying. Michael took the phone from Laura and, when he said 'hello,' John was on the other line.

"Michael, please keep us posted. Remember that we are your friends."

"I will do that, John."

"I have to hang up. I have to console Laura. Bye."

Michael hugged his wife. "Laura, you really surprised me. I thought you had cried enough since the diagnosis."

"I just could not help it. Every time I think about all the possible complications and opportunistic diseases that you might get afflicted with, I cry. I guess I am trying to picture you as the AIDS patients I have seen in the hospital. I am sorry, Michael. I will try to control my emotions better."

"Laura, it is not good to repress your emotions. That's how people really get ulcers and become depressed. It is better to cry. It makes you feel better."

"Thank you, Michael. Do you want to eat dinner?"

"I think I will just eat the dessert which Mom sent with us."

"How about coffee?"

"That would be fine, Laura. Thanks."

"We have to go to sleep early. I have big cases scheduled tomorrow, and I have to work at Southern Hospital."

"Laura, I thought you stopped moonlighting at Southern Hospital?"

"Michael, please, be realistic. I have to do it. We don't know how much you will get from your disability insurance. I am sure Dr. McIntyre will start you on AZT. AZT is so expensive."

"Dr. McIntyre said that he would ask the drug representative to give it to me at cost."

"I don't know whether this drug agent can do it for you. AZT is an orphan drug; that's why it is so expensive."

"I know, but there is no harm in asking."

"We will see what this drug agent says."

Laura woke up very early and left before Michael woke up. She had to finish her rounds before she went to the operating room. She might not have enough time to make rounds after surgery because she had to be at Southern Hospital by six-thirty in the evening.

Laura spent the whole day scrubbed in the operating room. With the first case, she scrubbed with the senior resident. A 54-year-old patient had been operated on four times for intestinal obstruction because of talc. She had developed more adhesions in the past six months.

"This is frustrating. I wish the drug companies would discover an agent to prevent adhesions."

"I wish so, too. I hope this patient does not come back before I finish my senior year."

"Well, I hope she does not come back during my senior year."

"Let's close while we are ahead."

Laura finished closing the incision. The senior resident went to the next room to do a breast biopsy with frozen section. In between cases, Laura tried to call Michael. Their phone was busy.

Laura went to her next case. It was a cholecystectomy with exploration of the common bile duct. The procedure went smoothly, and she was finished with this case in two hours. It helped that the patient was well-built and not obese.

Laura tried to call Michael again. "Michael, how are you? Did you eat the hot breakfast I prepared for you?"

"Yes, thank you. My T-cells are less than 500 per cubic mm. of blood. I have to take AZT, 100 mg for five doses, every four to five weeks. My blood has to be monitored, too. The AZT will depress my immune system and bone marrow."

"We have to switch to a macrobiotic diet. I bought a recipe book. There are some special recipes included in this book which I think you might like to try."

"Whatever you say, Laura. I have already taken the AZT that Dr. McIntyre had given me. This will be enough for the first course."

"Well, Michael, eat well and take care. I might not be able to call you again today unless I am not busy at Southern Hospital."

"Bye, I love you."

"I love you, too."

Laura rushed to Southern Hospital. By the time she arrived, the accident ward was jammed. There were several pregnant patients that had to be admitted to the delivery room immediately. She saw her first patient in room one. It was a 35-year-old lady, a rehabilitated drug addict, who had decided to go back to drugs. She had partied the whole night three days ago. She had injected cocaine in her umbilicus.

"How could you inject cocaine in your umbilicus? Suppose you hit some blood vessels in that area? You could have killed yourself!"

"Doctor, do your job. Stop lecturing me."

"Excuse me, I am just trying to educate you for your own welfare."

"I don't need a lecture from you."

"You need to be admitted for incision and drainage of this abscess. I have to call the surgeon-on-call here."

"I am signing out."

"Well, if you sign out, you will really be risking your life. You can die from overwhelming infections. You need to be started on intravenous antibiotics even before the surgeon can drain the abscess."

"How long do I have to stay in this hospital?"

"I can't answer that. It depends on the surgeon who operates on you."

"Can you tell him I want to stay only for one day?"

"No, that would be his decision."

"Well, I will stay. Who will be my doctor?"

"I will try to find out. I will have to call him. Just relax. I will take care of what is needed to get you admitted. I hope you will not try self-injection of cocaine again."

"I won't. Thank you."

Laura was quite busy at Southern Hospital. She did not have a chance to call Michael again.

Michael fell asleep while he was reading and was awakened by the phone ringing.

Ring===Ring===Ring

"Hello, Michael, it's Jorge. How are you holding up? Dr. Simmons gave us a call three days ago. I am sorry to hear the news. How is Laura taking this?"

"Well, she is taking it better than I. She is still working hard. She had to go back moonlighting at Southern Hospital. She is trying to save money for my medication, AZT. I started taking it today. But my doctor, Dr. McIntyre, gave me some which would take care of the first course of therapy. My healthcare insurance and disability will be covered for another year as stipulated in my contract. I wish this medicine would help delay the progress of my disease. I know I will never see Jennifer grow up. I leave everything in the hands of God. He knows what is best for all of us. Laura is so optimistic that I am afraid she does not realize that I might have a variant of AIDS with different manifestations from those that we usually see in the hospital, like cough, weight loss, night sweats, and tunnelling ulcers. I am afraid that I might be afflicted with a fatal type of AIDS that has a relatively short course. I have not even lost weight yet. My appetite is still good. I am just frustrated that I cannot work, even if I don't have patient contact. There is no research position available in the University for me. I am thinking of volunteering as a speaker for AIDS and being an AIDS buddy. I hope I will be able to do this. I don't like sitting in the apartment reading and sleeping while Laura is working two jobs so we can survive. I feel terrible. She should be depending on me, not the other way around. I can't take this any longer! I want to do things for other people. If I cannot be of use anymore as a practicing physician, I would at least like to be a volunteer and help educate people about AIDS and its prevention. I would like to help healthcare workers who might be afflicted with AIDS know more about protecting themselves against medical bureaucracy. I would like them to know how they can protect themselves through coverage of healthcare benefits once they are afflicted. All residents, interns, and fellows should be entitled to continuous healthcare benefits and disability benefits even if their contract is only for a year."

"Michael, your intentions are noble. I could not agree more with you. When a physician is afflicted with AIDS, he loses not only his career but his entire future and life. He should be entitled to a life insurance. Insurance companies would probably pay some of the money in advance when you need it for medical care."

"That's an idea worth pursuing, Jorge. How are Estela and Nedda doing?"

"They are doing fine. Estela went home for a visit to the Pineapple Republic. Her cousin Ditas might come back here to get a modeling job. A rich American lawyer and a Florida physician have been recruiting models there. They are supposed to use the models in their weight-reducing and work-out franchise. I don't know why they have to go to the Pineapple Republic to do this, though."

"Jorge, don't be naive. These guys are after cheap labor. They are recruited as tourists; therefore, they do not have to buy them health insurance. No life insurance and no disability insurance. Estela's cousin will have no leverage either. She will have only a tourist visa. I hope she is not gullible enough to believe these guys."

"Thank you for telling me, Michael. I better call Estela and warn her. Michael, please call if there is anything we can do for you. Bye, and give my best to Laura."

CHAPTER XXVIII

On July 15, 1985, Laura came home quite late. Her surgical schedule had been quite hectic. By the time she arrived home, Michael had fallen asleep while watching television. Laura was getting ready to prepare a snack, when she noticed an open envelope on the dining table. It was from the Jelton Realty Corporation. She took out the letter inside. The letter inside read: "The Jelton Realty Corporation wishes to inform you that, effective August 15, 1985, your month-to-month lease will no longer be renewed. Feel free to call the office if you have any questions."

Laura took the letter and put it inside her purse. She woke up Michael. "How are you? How was your day? Did you read this letter from the realtors?"

"Yes, I did. I think what they are doing to us is terrible. How come all of a sudden our lease is not going to be renewed anymore?"

"I don't know. I'll have to call their office tomorrow. I am going to demand an explanation about why they will not be renewing our lease! Let's get something to eat."

"I don't feel like eating, Laura. I am very disturbed with other people's reaction to my illness. Do you think the realtor knows that I have AIDS? How did he find out? It is supposed to be confidential."

"I don't know, Michael. That is why I have to demand a reason for their action against us."

"Laura, please do not make waves. Philadelphia's residents are not yet educated enough about AIDS. And, for you to make such a demand will just be inviting unneeded, biased publicity. It could affect your job, too. People might think that you have it, too."

"Let them suspect as much as they want. They will have to prove it. Why do people treat victims of AIDS so shabbily? Don't they realize that anyone or everyone of us may get infected with it? The public needs more education about AIDS. How about those patients who get it because of blood transfusion? How about hemophiliacs who get transfused with AIDS-infected blood products and develop AIDS later? These people get it not through their choice, but through inadequate and still not perfected blood testings. How about a surgical resident who gets AIDS through the improperly manufactured, poor-quality gloves which are being used in the operating room and which are being bought by hospitals in order to save money? How will society treat these people then?"

"AIDS victims are lumped into one basket, no matter how they've incurred the disease. People see victims of AIDS through their tunnel vision. They have no sympathy or compassion. People believe AIDS can be only sexually transmitted, and this belief lessens their sympathy for AIDS victims."

"Michael, it is getting late. We better go to sleep. I will be very busy tomorrow, but I want to call the realtor myself."

"Thanks, Laura."

Laura left very early. She fixed Michael a hot breakfast before she left. By the time she arrived at the hospital, the emergency room trauma center was overcrowded. There was a man who had gone berserk and had shot four people at a fast food store. Two of the victims were dead on arrival. The other two victims would have to be taken to the operating room and explored. One of them had a bullet wound in his head; the other one had been shot in the neck. The neurosurgeon and the cardiothoracic surgeon had to be called for the two patients. Laura was asked to assist on the neck case. On the way to the operating room, the patient suddenly stopped breathing in spite of being intubated. Laura was beside herself.

"Oh, my God, this is so catastrophic! The family of this man doesn't even know that he has been shot! How do you tell the family?"

The senior resident assigned Laura to look for the family in the emergency room. If she could not find them there, she was to call the policeman who had brought in the shooting victims, so he could go to their house and tell them to go to Northend Hospital. Laura went to the accident ward, but the family of John Steer was nowhere to be found.

In the meantime, the other patient with the head wound went into delirium tremens during induction of anaesthesia; he aspirated and unfortunately died, too. The neurosurgeon instructed the police to fetch the victim's family from home. He wanted to explain to the family what had happened inside the operating room.

The scenes in both the emergency and operating rooms were morbid. It was like being in the valley of death. There was such a somber silence that they could even hear the footsteps of people walking in the accident ward. Everyone felt very sad. Lives had been wasted needlessly because the mental health system had failed. The man who had gone berserk had just been discharged from a mental institution. He was supposed to have been stable.

Laura was exhausted before she even started her first case in the morning. All the scheduled operating room cases had to be moved back. The surgical schedule had to be changed. The Journal Club scheduled for that day had to be canceled. Laura did not get home until about 10:00 p.m.. She did not have the heart to wake up Michael when she got home. Laura's tears welled up in her eyes. Michael looked haggard, exhausted, and pale in spite of the rest he got everyday. His face looked sad and pained. Laura stroked Michael's hair and forehead. She could not help sobbing.

Michael woke up and asked, "What happened, Laura. Why are you crying?"

Laura just looked at Michael. "I am sorry, Michael; I just cannot help but cry. I am sorry that I did not have the chance to call the realty corporation either. I will do it tomorrow."

"Don't worry, Laura. We still have twenty-nine days left before they can throw us out."

The next morning, Laura woke up exhausted. Her eyes were red and swollen from crying all night. It had finally sunk into her last night what the letter from the realtor meant. But everything was happening too fast! She was still crying when she left for work. Her tears so blurred her driving that she would have had a bad accident, had it not been for the alert driver ahead of her. As it was, she had hit the car in front of her. Laura got out of her car to see if she had damaged the taillight of the car ahead of her.

When the man left his car and saw Laura, he felt sorry for her. "You look so tired and frightened. I think you better go home, rest, and get some sleep."

"I am just going to work, sir, but thank you for your concern. I was up all night trying to figure out what to do with our problems. My husband is sick and I am trying to work two jobs."

"Don't worry about the tiny dent. That's no problem. Here's my card if you ever need my help."

Laura took the card and put it inside her wallet. The nice, distinguished looking man left. Laura said to herself, "I am glad that there are still some decent people left in the world."

It was already nine o'clock when Laura arrived at the hospital. She had to call the realtor. Laura dialed the realtor's office. The manager spoke to her.

"Dr. Secula, did you receive our letter?"

"Yes, and it is extremely cut and dry. You gave us no explanation why our lease is being terminated."

"Well, we are going to upgrade and renovate the building, with each apartment being done one at a time. Since you are the only tenants with a month-to-month lease renewal, we decided to start the renovation with your apartment. We can give you another week's extension. After that, we will have no choice but to evict you."

"How can you do this to us? Are you sure there is no other reason other than the renovation?"

"I am positive."

"But this is so sudden!"

"It is not; it is a month's notice."

"Thank you for explaining the situation to me, but I am not convinced."

"I don't have to convince you, Dr. Secula. I just have to notify you of the expected change."

"Well, I am not going to take any more of your time. I have to make arrangements and look for another apartment. Thank you."

Laura was in tears when she hung up. "My God, please give us the courage and strength to overcome all our problems." She tried to call her mom, but her phone was busy. She finally talked to Mrs. Secula in the afternoon.

"Mom, how are you? How is Jennifer doing?"

"We are all doing fine. How about you and Michael?"

Laura paused, "Mom, may I call you back? I have to go to my call room. I have to ask you a favor. I will call you back in a minute."

As soon as Laura reached her room, she called back Mrs. Secula.

"Mom, we will not have a place to live after the middle of next month. We just received a letter from the realtor two days ago that our lease is being terminated. They gave us a one-week extension. What are we going to do? We don't have the kind of money for a security deposit and for one month's advance rent. We have more bills than I can handle."

"Laura, don't worry yourself to death. Michael and you can always move back with me and Jeanie. That would even be better for all of us. Michael and you will be with Jennifer most of the time. Michael will also be entertained by Jennifer's new motor development. She does something new practically everyday. It would be my pleasure and Jeanie's to have all of us together again."

"Mom, may I suggest something?"

"Sure."

"Mom, probably it would be much better that Michael and I live in the basement so that you and Jeanie don't lose your privacy."

"Whatever you want to do, but the basement needs remodeling."

"I will try to get a loan for the remodeling. We need a bathroom, and the patio would have to be enclosed."

"I will go along with that."

"Mom, can you do me a favor? Can you ask your neighbor who did her patio? We can probably use him, too."

"I will do that as soon as I hang up."

Laura tried to call several banks to see where she could take out a loan. Finally, she decided to go to a bank close to where her Mom lived.

Laura had a hard time filling out the application form. There were so many questions. She requested to talk to the manager of the bank so that she could explain her financial situation. She had loans to pay for both her and Michael's medical schooling, and for her car. She was still paying rent on the apartment and would soon be footing the bill for Michael's medications. On those bases alone, her loan was denied by the manager. She could not understand it; she was a responsible person, and she moonlighted extra days to enable her to keep up with their bills! The manager told her that, since her mother was the owner of the house, she should co-sign the loan. Laura was very frustrated. She did not realize that, when there was only one bread winner, life could be very tough and cruel. She went to her mother's house to ask her if she would co-sign the loan. Jennifer hugged her mommy and pulled her long hair; Laura was very happy to see Jennifer enjoying her stay with her Grandmom.

"Laura, do you want something to eat?"

"Mom, before anything else, I have to ask you another favor. The bank will not give me a loan unless you co-sign it, since you are the owner of the house being renovated."

"No problem, Laura. I will just give Jennifer her bottle, and then we will go to the bank with you."

Laura hugged her mom, "Thank you, Mom. I don't know what I would do without you and Jeanie."

"We are a family, Laura."

"Thanks, Mom."

Mrs. Secula prepared Jennifer's formula. She wanted to be sure that Jennifer did not miss any of her scheduled feedings.

Mrs. Secula and Laura went directly to the manager of the Kalina St. Bank as soon as they arrived. The manager was nice although he was a little hesitant to give Laura the loan even though her mom would co-sign it.

"Dr. Secula, I am doing this for you because I feel that you are a responsible person and that you will do your best to pay this loan on time. Otherwise, as I am sure you're aware, you will be jeopardizing your mom's financial situation."

"I understand completely what my responsibilities are. I assure you that the loan will be paid on time. Thank you."

Mrs. Secula, Laura, and Jennifer went back to the Secula residence. As soon as they got home, Laura went to the bathroom and started sobbing.

"I did not realize that being poor could be so humiliating and that a major family illness could tear you apart. Mom, I am just so thankful Michael and I have you and all our friends. It must be devastating for other families whose loved ones become ill and who have no one to turn to. Michael and I are really blessed in a very special way."

Mrs. Secula hugged Laura. "I am so proud of you for being so strong, for being so hopeful, and, most of all, for having such great faith in God. Your father would have been proud of you, too."

"I always feel that God is fair and that whatever misfortunes Michael and I are experiencing have happened for a reason. God does things in strange ways some times. Some misfortunes open up opportunities; some make you a stronger person and help you grow up emotionally, intellectually, and spiritually."

"Laura, I am so glad you feel that way. It makes me feel that I have raised the best daughter a mother could ever hope to nurture."

"Thanks, Mom."

"Let's call the contractor and ask him when he can come and start the job. You should be getting the check in three days."

"I hope so."

Laura called the contractor. He would not be able to come until Friday. Laura was on call at Southern Hospital on that day.

"My mother will explain the floor plan which I have sketched. If you can't understand my sketch, you can call me at the hospital. I hope you will give me a good price; I need a break."

"I will give you the best price around. You can compare my price with your neighbors. They all know me. I will be talking to you soon."

"Thank you."

Laura was getting ready to leave when Jennifer started crying. Laura took her from Mrs. Secula to see if her diaper was wet. Everything was fine with Jennifer except that she probably missed her mom and dad.

"Jennifer, Mommy has to go back home to see how Daddy is doing. Mommy and Daddy will come and see you Saturday."

Laura gave Jennifer to Mrs. Secula to hold. Laura could not help but cry on her way home. She missed Jennifer, too, but she had no choice. If only Jennifer could understand that her father was fighting for his life, she would know why her mom and dad couldn't have her with them.

By the time Laura arrived home, Michael was on the phone. He had gotten in touch with the AIDS hotline in the city. He would be doing volunteer work by phone. He would talk to other AIDS-afflicted people by phone.

Michael noticed that Laura's eyes were red and swollen.

"Laura, I know you must have been crying the whole afternoon. I wish you would share your thoughts with me. I know I can't be of much help physically, but emotionally and intellectually I might be of some use."

"You are, Michael. You have shown it to me in the way you have accepted God's will. I have a hard time accepting that we might have only a few months or years together. I have not really accepted the fact that I might lose you suddenly and that I might have to raise Jennifer all by myself."

"Laura, when someone dies, he does not really die. He goes to a better place where he can watch all the people he loves from above. Actually, death is a temporary separation from all the people one loves. Life on earth is only transient. Death does not destroy a person, but gives that person a better life and the ability to watch over his or her loved ones."

"Michael, I can't believe what I am hearing. I feel you are actually reciting a psalm for me."

"Laura, even when I am gone, I will always watch over you and Jennifer. I know you will try your best to raise Jennifer the way we were raised."

Laura started sobbing, "Michael, please don't talk like that. You don't even have any manifestations of AIDS so far."

"Laura, I am not sure how long it will take before the AIDS virus will overwhelm my immune system. I am hoping I will see Jennifer walk before my disease becomes terminal."

Laura hugged Michael.

"Michael, I am so proud of you. I wish I could think the way you do. I am really trying. I hope I am not upsetting you."

"Laura, you are reacting just as any loving wife would. I would be upset if you did not show any emotion at all!"

"Thank you, Michael. I will try my best not to get too emotional."

"No, Laura. You have to cry if you feel like crying. I don't want you to get an ulcer on top of everything else. I just want you to be realistic."

"I am trying my best, Michael."

"I know." Michael tried to wipe Laura's tears.

"I think I better cook dinner. Michael, why don't you turn on the news?"

Michael went to the living room and turned on the television. To his surprise, Debbie was being interviewed on the news.

"Laura, Laura, hurry up!"

"Why?"

"Debbie is being interviewed on T.V. about the increase in the number of homeless people with AIDS."

"Did she say how many have died?"

"Yes, twenty-two including Charlie Singleton."

"Did she say anything more?"

"No, they are just puzzled why all these homeless people are dying from AIDS."

"I wish someone would nail Robert Smith soon."

"Laura, you cannot just nail someone like Robert Smith. Hard evidence against him is needed."

"What more evidence do the authorities need? What better evidence is there than all those AIDS-infected victims of his lying in pain, emaciated, withdrawn, broken in spirit, awaiting their Maker with no one to look after them but the state? Sometimes even the state refuses to take care of its poor, sick, and homeless. The city doesn't care either. There is not much funding coming from the city."

"I know. The public is too apathetic and unaware of the situation."

"Until their family is stricken with AIDS, people just refuse to acknowledge the fact that AIDS does not discriminate. One can get it accidentally the way you did. Every healthcare worker is at risk of AIDS. I wish the healthcare authorities would find better ways of protecting healthcare workers. Cost-containment is not helping either. Latex gloves alone are supposed to protect people from AIDS, but, because of increased demand with less supply, gloves are being manufactured with no stringent quality control. I notice in the operating room that gloves tear very easily. By the time I am finished with one case, I have already used four pairs of gloves. Actually, it is not saving money at all."

"I agree with you. The quality of gloves is inferior."

"The attending physicians advise us to use two gloves every time we scrub. But it is very hard to operate that way. It limits my manual dexterity."

"I can understand what you mean. Just be careful when you scrub in the operating room. Jennifer needs one of us. Be careful when you tie with that Dexon suture. It is like a saw."

"I know. Thank you. Michael, dinner will be ready shortly. Actually, some of the food came from Mom. How do you want your steak?"

"Medium."

"Do you want mashed potatoes and mushrooms?"

"That would be fine."

"Orange juice or milk?"

"I think I will have orange juice."

"I will have to heat the dessert which Mom gave us."

When Michael and Laura sat down for dinner, the phone rang. Laura picked up the phone.

"Hello?"

"Laura, this is Jay Simmons. How are you? How is Michael doing?"

"Dr. Simmons, I will let you talk to Michael. We are doing fine. We just saw Debbie's T.V. interview tonight. She looked great! I am sure she is enjoying her new job. Please say 'hello' to her for us. Here's Michael."

"Thank you, Laura."

Michael took the phone from Laura.

"Dr. Simmons, how are you? Thank you for thinking of us."

"Michael, I think it is time for your repeat blood count. I can take you to the hospital tomorrow. I will pick you up at eight o'clock and we can both have breakfast at the cafeteria. What do you think?"

"That is a good idea. We can probably inquire if there is an opening at the research department of the university hospital."

The next morning, Laura left very early. She had been assigned to report to the Surgical Journal Club. By the time she arrived at the hospital, there was a big commotion in the accident ward. A 16-year-old girl was being resuscitated. She was found hemorrhaging in the bathroom. She was supposed to have had an abortion two days ago at the Wobble Abortion Clinic. The patient was bleeding throughout all her cavities. O negative blood was pumped into her to no avail. After one and a half hours of failed heroic measures, she was pronounced dead. The coroner's office was notified. The grief-stricken mother became hysterical.

"I am going to sue that clinic and all the damn abortionists there! They killed my daughter and her baby! I did not even know she went to the clinic."

Laura called Debbie at the Coroner's office.

"Debbie, how are you?"

"I am fine, thank you. How is Michael doing?"

"He is the same, but a little bit more pale and haggard."

"What can I do for you, Laura?"

"We have a young girl in the accident ward who came here practically bled out. She was supposed to have had an abortion. Her mother did not know anything about it until she found her hemorrhaging in the bathroom."

"This is terrible!"

"Moreover, she used somebody else's medical assistance card to pay for the abortion."

"I will call the D.A.'s office if I feel criminal charges should be filed against the doctor. Was she seen in another emergency room before she came to yours?"

"Yes, she went to Southern Hospital for vaginal spotting, but was not admitted because she did not have money, a Medicaid card, or any other insurance."

"This is atrocious!"

"I know."

"I will call you as soon as I get the final report of the autopsy."

"Thank you, Debbie. Give my love to your dad."

"I will do that. Bye."

On her way to the Journal Club, Laura was paged by the operator.

"Hello, may I help you? I am Dr. Secula."

"This is the manager of Kalina St. Bank. I am sorry, but we can't approve your loan with only your mother as the co-signer. She is on a fixed income, and with real estate tax being increased every year, she might not be able to help you out. Do you have any relative who has a stable job?"

"Yes, my sister."

"She can probably co-sign it for you."

"I will call her and let you know."

"Thank you."

After she hung up, Laura went up to her room and started crying. She dialed her mom's number.

"Mom, this is Laura. My loan application was not approved."

"Laura, calm down, calm down. I will give you Jeanie's number. Call her at work and ask her to co-sign for you."

"Thanks, Mom."

Laura called Jeanie at work.

"Laura, why do you sound so distraught? Did something happen to Michael?"

"No, Jeanie. I need your help. My loan was not approved. I need another loan co-signer."

"Laura, you know I will do that for you. We are a family. Who else but family will help one of its own?"

"Will you be able to go to the bank and sign some papers?"

"Sure, I will get an extra hour for lunch today and drive to the bank then."

"Thank you, Jeanie. Michael and I are coming down tomorrow night. We miss Jennifer so much."

"I understand. We will see you tomorrow then. Bye."

Laura started crying again after she hung up. "Thank God I have a nice, loving family."

Laura missed the Journal Club. She went directly to the operating room to scrub with the first year resident on a case of intestinal obstruction. The obstructed patient had been admitted from the accident ward eight hours ago. He had been vomiting several hours prior to admission and had been constipated for the last two weeks. He also had emphysema due to chain smoking for twenty years. He was a very poor anaesthetic risk. His wife, who brought him in, was told of all the possible complications of surgery and anaesthesia.

"I have no choice but to co-sign this permit and informed consent. I know that surgery is the only solution for his problem. I am well aware that he could die on the operating table."

"Thank you for your understanding, Mrs. Small. It makes our job a little bit easier," said Laura.

"Where do I stay while you are operating?"

"You can wait in the patient's lounge. I will come down as soon as the operation is over."

Laura and the senior resident did an exploration on Mr. Small. On opening his abdomen, they noticed a huge, cauliflower-like mass that had invaded the whole length of the large bowel.

"Laura, we can't do anything for this patient. We might as well close the abdomen. We cannot even mobilize the colon to do a colostomy. Everything is matted together."

"Poor soul. How do I tell Mrs. Small now? This poor lady was expecting us to at least alleviate her husband's symptoms. She has no idea that her husband's surgical condition is quite advanced."

"Well, we just have to tell her the truth."

"I will do that."

As soon as the operation was over, Laura went down to the patient's lounge to talk to Mrs. Small. Laura took Mrs. Small aside.

"Mrs. Small, I am very sorry to tell you, but we could not do much for Mr. Small. All the bowels were matted together by cancer cells. It would have jeopardized his life if we had tried to do more. We can at least make him comfortable with pain medications for the rest of his life. I know it is easier for me to say this since it's the patient himself who is feeling the pain. I can sympathize with you, though; my husband is very sick, too. Please do not hold your tears back. Cry. It will make you feel better, and it will make you feel more human. Crying is your only outlet against depression and frustration."

Laura squeezed Mrs. Small's hand tightly and said, "You are not alone. If you feel like talking, please feel free to call me."

"Thank you, Dr. Secula."

Laura went back to her call room before going to the cafeteria for lunch. The anchor of the afternoon news on T.V. said, "An HMO doctor lost a breast case for three million dollars. Dr. Dough lost a medical malpractice suit filed against him by the estate of a deceased patient whose bilateral breast cancer was ignored by him deliberately because of financial incentive. HMO paid two million dollars, and the employer paid one million dollars."

Laura quickly called Michael.

"How are you? Did you enjoy the breakfast I cooked for you?"

"Naturally, I just love pancakes."

"Guess what?"

"What, Laura?"

"Dr. Dough was on T.V. this afternoon. He lost a bilateral breast case to the family of a 29-year-old lady who died two years ago."

"I know. I just heard it in the news. I want to know more about the case."

"I'll try to get the night edition of the *Philadelphia Gazette* before I come home today. I have to hang up now. I have a few more minor cases before my surgical clinic today."

"I will see you tonight."

"Take care, Michael. Do you want me to get something from the grocery?"

"We do not need anything right now. Bye, don't work too hard."

Laura picked up the *Philadelphia Gazette* evening edition in the hospital lobby before she went home. The gazette contained an interview of the plaintiff lawyer. Mrs. Sinclair, who left two young children, ages three and four, was forced to join HMO through her husband's job. The company offered *only* one type of insurance, HMO. She was assigned to Dr. Dough. Mrs. Sinclair went to Dr. Dough complaining of breast tenderness and bilateral lumps.

"These are only cysts, Mrs. Sinclair."

"But I can feel lumps on both my breasts."

"Well, come back in six months. I will recheck you. If you feel a lot of pain, use this Nupercaine Cream."

"I am worried about my breasts, Dr. Dough. Cancer of the breast runs in my family."

"You are too young for that. Come back in six months. Besides, according to the HMO guideline, mammography should be done only at age forty."

Thus had the plaintiff lawyer repeated to the jury what Mrs. Sinclair had told him before she died about that fateful conversation with Dr. Dough. He also showed them a video of two sad children playing in their backyard and asking questions such as, "Where is mommy? How come she is not here to play with us? How come we don't see our mommy? How come other kids have mommies to play with, to swim with, and to take them to school? How come mommy does not go to church with us?"

Michael and Laura both broke down while reading the newspaper account. The content of the interview was too close to home. They both continued reading.

"The HMO insurance was sued, too, because Dr. Dough was the agent of HMO. HMO appealed the verdict on the basis of the hold harmless clause, but lost. The employer was successfully sued, too, because offering only an HMO insurance is illegal according to the HMO Federal Act of 1973," stated the plaintiff lawyer.

"Every dog has its day. More power to the lawyer who vigorously pursued Dr. Dough, the HMO, and the employer. Everyone should be made accountable for trying to set the trend of medical practice, including employers!" said Michael.

Ring===Ring===Ring===Ring

Laura went to the kitchen to answer the phone. It was Jeanie.

"Laura, I co-signed the loan today, and the bank manager said you can pick up the check tomorrow."

"Jeanie, thank you so much! May I talk to Mom?"

Jeanie handed the phone to her mother.

"Mom, thanks to both of you. Could you please call the contractor tomorrow to see when he can start the renovation?"

"I will gladly call him tomorrow. Jennifer is sleeping in my arms now. She was very tired today."

"At least I will be able to spend more time with Jennifer once we move there. Michael will be able to play with her everyday. That will help Michael keep his mind off his illness. Jennifer will be his therapy, too."

"I am looking forward to having you all here."

"Good night, Mom. Do you want to talk to Michael?"

"Yes."

Laura handed the phone to Michael.

"Mom, thank you so much for all your moral support and for taking care of Jennifer. We look forward to moving in with you. Jennifer must keep you busy the whole day."

"Don't worry, Michael. I love every minute of it. Jennifer keeps me young with her new antics every day."

"Good night, Mom." Laura started packing when Michael finished talking to Mrs. Secula.

"Michael, I think we better start packing our books. Please put all your florigraphy books in a separate box and mark the florigraphy book that has in it Charlie's two letters to you."

"I will do that, Laura."

"I have to leave early for work tomorrow. Our surgical grand round starts at seven in the morning. I want to make rounds before the meeting starts. Our surgical schedule is quite heavy. We have about four major cases. I might not be able to call you tomorrow between operating cases. Please call Mom to see if she was able to get the contractor. I hope he will finish the renovation before our lease extension expires."

"I hope so, too. Laura, please get some sleep now. I am just going to finish packing all these books. I will be fine. Don't worry about me."

"But at least if I am awake, you will have someone to talk to."

"Thanks, Laura."

CHAPTER XXIX

Laura woke up very early. By the time she arrived at Northend Hospital, there was hardly a parking space left. She rushed to the ward so that she could discharge some of the patients whose sutures had to be removed. By seven o'clock, the grand round started. The first case was 29-year-old lady with gastric cancer. The patient's gastric symptoms were aggravated during pregnancy as severe intractable hyperemesis gravidarum. After the termination of pregnancy was accomplished, her gastric symptoms became worse. An upper G.I. was done and revealed the presence of a cancerous lesion in the greater curvature of the stomach.

"What is the lesson you can learn from this case?" asked Dr. Saltine.

Laura responded, "Not all cases of hyperemesis gravidarum are due to pregnancy alone. Never presume; always investigate the cause of pernicious vomiting in pregnancy."

"Do each and everyone of you agree?"

"Absolutely," the residents responded in unison.

After the grand round, all the residents proceeded to the operating room for their respective operations. Laura called Michael between cases. Their phone was busy. Laura presumed Michael was talking to fellow AIDS victims.

By five o'clock, Laura was getting ready to leave when she got a phone call.

"Hello, this is Laura Secula."

"Laura, this is Debbie. I just finished the autopsy on that 16-year-old girl."

"What did you find?"

"Well, I am very disturbed with my gross findings. There was perforation of the uterus and there was an ectopic pregnancy on the right cornual area which ruptured and caused the hemorrhage, thereby killing the patient. I have no choice but to tell the parents about my findings. Moreover, Southern Hospital might be slapped with a federal offense suit and a fine of $50,000.00 for not admitting the patient because she had no insurance. This suit will be under the COBRA law. This type of lawsuit will rise in the 90's because of cost-containment and the survival factor for the hospital and doctors. All the plaintiff lawyer has to do is incorporate these lawsuits with medical malpractice lawsuits. The family is planning to sue the Wobble Abortion Clinic, too, for fraud."

"How do they intend to prove fraud?"

"There was no informed consent, and the patient did not understand the risks involved. Nobody explained to her that she could die as a result of this operation."

"Well, abortion is a big business. The public has been successfully kept in the dark about the medical and surgical risks of abortion. The way it is being played up in the newspapers and television, it is just an innocuous procedure. We both know that this is a major misconception on the part of the public."

"The family is also planning to sue the abortionist for medical malpractice and fraud, along with the clinic."

"Do you think it is possible to sue for fraud under the Pennsylvania law?"

"Someone has to start it sometime. Fraud has been successfully used many times in medical malpractice in other states. Pennsylvania should get its first test case soon."

"I agree with you. There should be justice and fairness for everyone."

"I hope you realize that Southern Hospital might get bankrupt as a result of this incident. Sixty-five percent of their patients are on Medicare. The medicare contract of the hospital will be suspended for a period of time. Even though the emergency ward is a separate profit-making corporation, the hospital will still be liable."

"Do whatever you have to do, Debbie. I can always find a moonlighting job."

"Laura, the causes of all these problems in the healthcare crisis are greed, selfishness, and materialism. People are being damaged unnecessarily and sometimes are even dying needlessly. These problems have to be solved."

"How do you solve the multitude and magnitude of these problems?"

"By praying. There should be a Prayer for America Campaign nationwide. God is already chastising us for our warped moral and spiritual values. All these hurricanes might just be warnings. There might be worse things to come. God did it in Chernobyl to warn the Russians."

"I know, the message of the Blessed Virgin seems very urgent. She has appeared to the visionaries in Medjugorje a thousand times. We need to bring God to ourselves in our daily lives."

"I cannot agree more. Laura, I have to hang up now. Please give my love to Michael."

"I will. Thank you for your concern."

Laura went home, really upset about the 16-year-old girl who had died needlessly.

She raced over the expressway and got home in no time. While she was waiting for the elevator, she saw a girl who used to work at Dr. Tearcell's office. Laura said hello to her, but the girl completely ignored her, and went inside the manager's office. Laura was floored.

"Is she responsible for the termination of our lease?" Laura asked herself.

As soon as she entered their apartment, she blurted to Michael, "I know why our lease was suddenly terminated!"

"Why?"

"I have a sneaking suspicion that the secretary of Dr. Tearcell must have something to do with it."

"How do you know?"

"She works in the building now as the manager. She completely ignored me when I said 'hello'."

"Laura, this might just be coincidence."

"It is too obvious just to be a coincidence."

"If she did, then she violated the trust of Dr. Tearcell."

"I know and Dr. Tearcell does not even know anything about it. That is really a shame."

"There is nothing we can do about it. We cannot go public. People are not educated enough about AIDS yet to understand our predicament."

"I know."

"Laura, please turn the T.V. on."

"Which channel do you want?"

"It does not matter."

Laura turned on the T.V. to Channel 9.

"Laura, come here. Debbie is on T.V. again."

"She is being interviewed about the 16-year-old who died of botched abortion."

"Dr. Simmons, is the D.A. going to file criminal charges against the doctor and the abortion clinic?"

"I don't know."

"Do you think this patient should have been admitted to Southern Hospital?"

"I am not in a position to answer the question. I did not have the chance to examine the patient while she was still alive."

"Thank you for your time, Dr. Simmons."

"You are welcome."

The next day, Laura saw a picture of Debbie in the *Philadelphia Gazette* which also ran the same T.V. interview.

Laura called Michael, "Debbie's picture is in the *Philadelphia Gazette.* She is now a big celebrity in Philadelphia. I am sure Dr. Simmons is very proud of her."

"I am sure he is. She is his daughter."

Laura and Michael went to visit Jennifer and Mrs. Secula. The renovation had just started. The contractor promised that the job would be finished on time. The carpets had to be ordered and the plumber had to install the bathroom. The patio would be enclosed with screen and vinyl siding with a reinforced heating system so that Michael could stay in the porch during winter time.

Mrs. Secula told Michael and Laura, "Everything is working out according to schedule. Mr. Winkus has been more than accommodating with this changed floor plan."

"We are grateful for that. We are looking forward to moving here on time."

"I am sure you will be moving on time."

Laura took Jennifer from Mrs. Secula. She put her on her lap.

"Jennifer, Mommy and Daddy will soon be staying with you permanently. You will be seeing Daddy everyday, and you will be able to play with him." Jennifer just smiled and cooed.

By ten o'clock, Jennifer was asleep. Laura and Michael drove home leisurely, both in deep thought.

"Michael, we should call Father John as soon as we arrive home."

"Why?"

"We have to tell him we are moving out in two weeks so he will know where to call us. He will probably want to visit us, too."

"I think you are right. I am sure he will be happy to hear from us."

Michael and Laura went up to their apartment. On the door, they found a note attached to the door-knob.

The note read, "Leave this building soon with your plague. You are a disgrace to this apartment community."

Laura grabbed the note from Michael.

"Don't let yourself get upset by the nasty comments of sick, uneducated people, Michael. It only shows how small they are. They don't even know how you got AIDS, and they have the gall to leave this letter on the door-knob! They should be ashamed of themselves! These people should have compassion in their hearts rather than hatred for fellow human beings in agony. They should look at themselves in the mirror and examine their own reflections. How judgmental can they be? I am sure they are not perfect either."

"I am quite positive they are not perfect."

"Michael, do you want something to eat before we go to bed?"

"I would like to drink warm milk."

Michael and Laura sat at the dining table for awhile and talked.

"I will start packing tomorrow. I can start packing our clothes and books."

"We will get a mover to handle all the boxes and furniture. I don't want you to do any heavy lifting. You look quite tired. Get some rest, Michael. Don't pack the whole day. As soon as you get tired, just relax and call your AIDS buddies. I know you have been calling some of your friends."

"I have been talking to them for the past several weeks. We try to encourage each other. I find it very uplifting to talk to fellow victims because I know I am not the only one with this unpredictable, ugly disease."

"Michael, I am very glad you are able to express your frustrations, hopes, and fears with your buddies. I am sure they must find your verbal interactions uplifting, too."

"I am positive."

"Let's go to bed. Good night, Michael."

Laura woke up very early. She would be presenting her operative cases at the grand round. As soon as she arrived at the hospital, she noticed the crowded accident ward. The mother of a 35-year-old lady who had expired from respiratory failure due to massive hydrothorax and ascites could not be calmed down. She was very upset and quite hysterical. Her daughter had just had a hysterectomy with removal of both tubes and ovaries in another hospital. The family was told that the pathology report was benign for all the reproductive organs removed. Her brother happened to be a doctor. He wanted to hire an independent toxicologist and an independent pathologist to do the autopsy and microscopic examinations of all the organs and tissues. What made her brother suspicious was that her CEA and CA 125 were both elevated one month after surgery. He also asked someone to review the gynecologic pathology slides and to do deeper cuts on the paraffin blocks and to do more cuts from the previously preserved hysterectomy specimens. He also asked that the pap smear slides from the cytology laboratory of the same hospital be reviewed.

The brother of the deceased, Dr. Kipple, said in anger, "Heads will roll if any doctor caused the death of my sister through negligence. They will all pay and they will pay big! I will never stop until I get their licenses taken away from them. I want them to be in the National Data Bank. I would work with any consumer group who would like this Data Bank made public from the conspiracy of silence in my own profession. We deserve what we are getting from the public. I have to put the medical profession on trial and bring it to its knees. It is time for the medical profession to take a long, hard look at itself."

Laura was stunned when she heard Dr. Kipple.

"My God, this doctor is out for the blood of the medical profession,"she thought. Laura just stood there and listened to what Dr. Kipple was saying.

"I am going to scrutinize the chart of my sister microscopically and see if all the preadmission testings were done accurately. I will also get all the copies of any Ultrasound or CAT Scan done on her. That chart better be in order! No one will be spared in this investigation! Some doctors want to play with lives and don't consult other doctors. One cannot know everything!"

Suddenly, Laura was paged for the floor. She left Dr. Kipple and hurried to the fourth floor. She completely had forgotten that she was in charge of the grand round.

"I am sorry, guys. I forgot all about the grand round. I was quite taken by the death in the accident ward of a 35-year-old lady with a metastic tumor."

"What happened?"

"Her brother, who is a doctor, just blasted and tore apart the medical profession. He is going to put conspiracy of silence on trial. He is going to get an independent pathologist and toxicologist from another state to perform the autopsy on his sister. He will have the gynecologic pathology slides and pap smear slides checked by an independent pathologist."

"It is good that he can afford this. How about the poor patient in the same circumstances whose family cannot afford an independent pathologist to do the autopsy?"

"The family will be at a disadvantage in trying to prove negligence, especially if the pathologist is not familiar with the disease the deceased had. Then the final report of the autopsy will be delayed for months and months. The slides will be sent to different pathologists in the country."

"As we all know, money talks."

"Do we all know that?"

"Laura, what happened to your lady with malignant melanoma?"

"She went home happy. She does not need any further treatment or medications. Guys, let's talk about prophylactic antibiotics in surgery. Are you all for it?"

"I am, but we must realize that there is risk with antibiotics, too, such as colitis, yeast infection, bone marrow depression, and prolonged bleeding time, etc."

"Well, the patient should be told the risks first and then told the risks of not giving prophylactic antibiotics."

"I like to do cultures and a gram stain before I start the antibiotic."

"That's not a bad idea."

"Well, we better go to the operating room now before our cases are canceled."

"Let's go."

Before Laura scrubbed, she called Michael. Their phone was busy. It was almost two o'clock when Laura finally finished in the operating room. She called Michael again. There was no answer. Laura went back to the operating room again to see if there was any message for her.

"Dr. Secula, your husband called while you were operating. He said that Dr. Simmons would be taking him to Dr. McIntyre for a check-up. He will call you as soon as he is back."

"Thank you. For a while I was worried. I thought something happened to him."

Michael called Laura around four o'clock. It was good news.

"I have no physical manifestations of AIDS at all. Dr. McIntyre wants to repeat my T-cell count before we move to Kalina St.. Dr. Simmons volunteered to take me to the hospital again."

"That's very nice of him. Michael, we have to call Fr. John as soon as I come home. He might want to come and visit us. This time nothing should stop us from calling him."

"I hope so. See you then."

Laura was home by six o'clock. She cooked dinner and, after dinner, Michael got on the phone to call Father John.

"Hello, Father John. This is Michael. How are you, Father?"

"I am fine. How are you and Laura doing?"

"We are both doing fine. Laura and I are moving back to Kalina St. within two weeks as soon as the renovation of the basement is finished. We hope you will be able to come and visit us."

"I thought I would be able to, but our fund-raising campaign is not over yet. I will visit you as soon as the campaign is over."

"We will be expecting you then. I will have Laura talk to you now."

"Bye, Michael."

"Good night, Father John."

"Father, how are you?"

"I am fine, Laura. How are you and Jennifer?"

"We are all fine. Michael just had his physical examination today. He is fine. He is going to have his T-cell count repeated before we move to Kalina St.. We will love to have you come and visit us as soon as possible. Jennifer is getting bigger and more mischievous. She keeps my mother young."

"I am sure she is quite a bundle of joy."

"Thank you, Father. We look forward to seeing you soon. Good night, Father."

After Laura got off the phone, she turned to Michael, "Now we can do some more packing before we go to sleep."

"I have already packed most of our clothes and books. We really have few things left to pack. We can do the rest two days before the movers come."

"That would be fine with me, Michael. I think I better call Mom to see when the basement will be finally finished."

Laura dialed her mother's number and got her mom right away.

"Mom, how are you all doing?"

"We are all fine. The work is on schedule. The contractor thinks he can finish the whole job by the end of next week. I will call the carpet installer Monday. The plumbing is all finished. You might even be able to move sooner than you thought."

"I am glad, Mom. Michael and I are tired of staying in this apartment. I see nasty notes on the door-knob every morning before I go to work. I don't even tell Michael anymore. I don't want to upset him anymore than is necessary. Nasty people have nothing more important to do than interfere with other people's lives."

"I agree with you about not telling Michael about all those nasty notes. Michael has had enough pain to deal with. He should not have to deal with people's nastiness as well. It just seems so cruel for people to even think of writing nasty notes."

"I know; some people are just so miserable and unhappy with themselves that they are unable to show kindness or compassion to anyone."

"I am glad you feel that way, Laura. I am so proud of you."

"Thanks, Mom. You always make me feel good about myself."

"That's what mothers are for. Let me talk to Michael."

Michael got on the phone. "Mom, thank you for all your support and kindness to me and Laura. You have been our tower of strength throughout this ordeal. God has been good to me and Laura. We are so lucky to have you around when we need you most. Dr. Simmons took me to Dr. McIntyre today. He gave me a good check-up. I will have to have some blood tests done before we move to Kalina St., though."

"I am glad to hear that, Michael. I have to get off now. Princess Jennifer has fallen asleep in my arms. You take care. I will be talking to you and Laura again. I hope you will be able to move here before your lease is terminated. Good night, Michael."

"Good night, Mom."

As soon as Michael hung up, the phone rang. It was Dr. Simmons.

"Michael, I just got a letter from our lawyer. Robert Smith wants to depose all of us in two months. So, I have to call James Dillon and John Miller. By that time, you and Laura will probably have moved to Kalina St.."

"That would be fine, Dr. Simmons. The sooner we do it, the better. This guy is really on a fishing expedition. I would like to meet Mr. Robert Smith soon. He might be the same Robert Smith who peddles drugs to homeless people downtown. It would be a turning pint in our case if he were. All we have to do is hire detectives to find out if he is the same Robert Smith who killed Charlie."

CHAPTER XXX

Laura was walking through the lobby of Northend Hospital on her way to the parking lot when she accidentally saw a copy of the *Philadelphia Gazette* on the information desk. The headline read: "Robert Smith, the eminent medical malpractice lawyer, lost his bid for municipal judgeship." Laura asked the permission of the receptionist to read her paper.

The lady nodded. "You may take it with you, doctor. I am done with it."

"Thank you very much. I think my husband will be interested in reading this article. Thank you for the paper."

"You're welcome, doctor."

Michael was on the phone with Mrs. Secula when Laura arrived home. Laura whispered to Michael that she wanted to talk to her mom.

"Mom, I will put Laura on. She wants to talk to you."

"Mom, how is Jennifer?"

"Jennifer is fine. She did well today. She started sitting up. She ate better today, too. Pretty soon, she will be walking!"

"I hope she does not tire you that much."

"Laura, I love every minute I spend with Jennifer. She keeps me active."

"How is the contractor doing?"

"I think you might be able to move sooner than I thought. The carpet installer is coming on Tuesday. The plumber is done. You might be able to move Friday or Saturday."

"I think it is better that we move on Saturday morning. I will be working at Southern Hospital on Thursday night."

"That is not a problem, Laura. It is up to you. You move whenever you are ready. Jeanie and I will be able to help you with your last minute packing."

"Thanks, Mom. Dr. Simmons will take Michael on Friday for his regular blood test. I am keeping my fingers crossed that his T-cells will be the same."

"I hope so, too."

Laura had just hung up when the phone rang again. It was Estela. She had just come back from the Pineapple Republic. Her cousin, Ditas, was soon to start working for an American lawyer and a doctor in a health-spa and weight-reducing center.

"Estela, what is the name of this lawyer?"

"I think it is Robert Smith."

"How about the doctor's name?"

"Dr. Samuel Greedy."

"Is Robert Smith from Florida?"

"I guess so. The business outfit is located in Florida."

"I see. How is Nedda? She must be big now."

"She is starting to unroll toilet paper, and she puts her toys all over the living room. She is two going on six."

"I can imagine!"

"How is Jennifer?"

"She is doing fine. She is staying with Mom right now. We are going to move back with Mom. We are going to stay in the basement apartment. The realtor terminated our lease. We do not know the real reason for the termination of our lease."

"I am sorry to hear that. Why don't you and Michael come down here for a vacation? The weather and sun here might be good for him."

"We cannot do that now. Michael is being monitored closely by Dr. McIntyre. So far his blood testings have been the same. He will get his blood test repeated on Friday. Dr. Simmons will drive him to the university. Debbie and Dr. Simmons have been very thoughtful. Please say 'hello' to Jorge for me."

"I will do that. As I have said before, you are always welcome to come down here for a vacation."

"Thank you, Estela."

As soon as Laura hung up, she handed the *Philadelphia Gazette* to Michael.

"Isn't this the same Robert Smith Charlie told you about? Also, think about this, Michael. Estela just told me her cousin will be working for a lawyer named Robert Smith down in Florida. There is a lot of drug dealing going on in Florida. Don't you think Charlie's Robert Smith and Ditas' future boss might be one and the same?"

"I don't know, Laura. There are about twenty lawyers in Philadelphia whose name is Robert Smith. So we better be careful. Another Robert Smith might hear what we are saying and might sue us for defamation of character."

"I know that, Michael. But are the four of you going to let this Robert Smith ridicule and abuse the legal process without launching an investigation of your own to see if he is connected in some way to Charlie's and maybe Ditas' Robert Smith?"

"I don't know, Laura. I have to talk to Dr. Simmons about this matter. I have to ask the opinion of James Dillon and Joe Miller, too. Let me read the newspaper first before I make any decision on what to do."

"I am sorry, Michael. I am just upset about his frivolous suit. I hope it will get resolved soon."

"You know, Laura, you might be right! It says here in the paper that this Robert Smith has an office in Florida! But we really have no way of being certain. Maybe, at the deposition, he might say something that will give us a better idea if he is Charlie's Robert Smith. We have to see."

"I hope so. It is getting late, Michael. You better rest. I know you feel very tired. I will just write up some medical reports. I will join you later."

The next morning, Laura woke up early. She heard a knock on the door. She opened the door and found another nasty note on the door-knob. "When will you move out of this apartment building, queers?" Laura's face was streaked with tears and anger.

"These people are so cruel and ignorant! How can they be so heartless?"

She put the note into her handbag. She did not want Michael to see it. She cooked breakfast for Michael and left after drinking coffee. She left a note for Michael to call her at work. She was worried she might not be able to call him from Southern Hospital that night.

Laura was in the operating room the whole day. She called Michael between cases, but the phone was busy. She decided to call him later in the afternoon. Michael finally answered.

"Laura, I hope you were not trying to call me. I fell asleep. I did not realize that the phone was off the hook."

"I did try to call you. I was quite worried that something happened to you. I am glad you are fine."

"Thank you. I called several of my AIDS buddies today. Each of them is doing well."

"I am glad you were able to talk to them. I hope you feel better when you know all your buddies are doing as well as you."

"I really do. I think just talking to them helps me emotionally, too."

"I am happy for you, too. Michael, I will see you tomorrow night. Don't forget your appointment with Dr. Simmons tomorrow."

"Don't work too hard, Laura."

"Take care, Michael. I will come home early tomorrow."

Laura rushed to Southern Hospital. She was passing by the Neonatal Intensive Care Unit when she noticed the neonatologist busy resuscitating a baby. She found out that this baby's mother had been afflicted with Lyme's disease during the first trimester of her pregnancy. The motor development of the boy was poor. The baby was also small for gestational age. The intravenous massive antibiotics did not spare the baby the devastating effects of Lyme's disease during the development and growth in utero during the first trimester. It was such a horrible disease to get during the first two trimesters of pregnancy! There was no reliable test available so far. A physician had to rely only on physical symptoms and signs which could mimic other diseases. Laura felt very sad when she found out how the baby's development in utero was affected. She thought of Jennifer.

"Thank God, Jennifer is healthy."

Laura became so preoccupied with the poorly developed baby that she called her mom.

"Mom, how is Jennifer?"

"Jennifer is fine and is about to go to sleep. She is tired today. How is Michael doing?"

"He is fine, but I think he feels very tired. I think it is his personal anguish of not being able to operate that makes him feel so tired. I can just see it in his eyes and in the way he stands and walks. I feel like crying every time I look at him. There is so much sadness in those big blue eyes. Sometimes, I cry in the bathroom. If I could only divide the sadness between the two of us, I would not feel this bad. He does not even complain. He has completely accepted God's will. His faith amazes me. He has so much love, caring, and compassion in his heart. He calls his AIDS buddies every day to see how they are coping; yet, he is trying to cope with the same disease himself. He is really bigger than life."

"Laura, don't feel bad. I know Michael is aware that you care about him. He has told me many times how lucky he is for having you as his wife."

"I know, Mom. But, sometimes I feel I married a saint."

Laura was busy in the accident ward. At twelve midnight, a pregnant lady with previous Caesarean section arrived in active labor and in shock. She immediately inserted an intravenous line, and typed and crossed four units of blood. O negative blood was pumped. The obstetrician was already waiting in the delivery room. By the time the woman got to the delivery room, the fetal heartbeat could not be heard. The fetal monitoring tracing showed no fetal cardiac activity. A crash induction was done. As soon as the abdomen was opened, the baby was found in the abdominal cavity, stillborn, with the bleeding, ruptured uterine scar. The patient's blood pressure suddenly dropped. Her cardiac rate went up to 200/minute. The bleeding branches of the uterine vessels could not be contained. The cardiac monitor showed ventricular tachycardia; then, all of a sudden, the patient started bleeding throughout all her cavities.

"My God, is this patient having incompatible blood transfusion reaction or uncontrollable hemorrhage?"

Code 1, DR Room Two===Code 1, DR Room Two

Everyone rushed to D.R. two. It was futile. The patient had died from cardiac arrest.

The obstetrician, Dr. McKinney, went out to the waiting room to explain to the family what had transpired in the delivery room.

"I don't know what to say. This is such a tragic situation. Your wife should have had a repeat Caesarean section electively. I am so furious with the insurance company and obstetrical consultant of the insurance company for turning down the request of your wife for an elective repeat Caesarean section."

"My wife insisted to the obstetrical consultant that she was afraid to go into labor. She had all these fears about going into labor and dying during labor. The obstetrical consultant would not even listen to her pleadings. He has no heart. He and the insurance companies should be made accountable. They both have conflict of interest. My wife's obstetrician even called the insurance company and the second opinion surgical consultant to no avail. My wife's obstetrician has that conversation well-documented on her chart. We were with him in the consultation room when he talked to the doctor and the utilization reviewer of the insurance company. He was livid."

"You have reason to go after them, and I am willing to support you. I have to call your wife's obstetrician now. Again, I am very sorry I was not able to help you. Please, feel free to call me."

Dr. McKinney called Dr. Kelvey.

"Dr. Kelvey, I am sorry to tell you that one of your patients died on the operating table for ruptured uterine scar and uncontrollable hemorrhage."

"Oh, my God! Gina never wanted a trial of labor. I pleaded with the insurance company and the second opinion consultant, but they would not listen to any of my medical reasons. I told them that she should not be allowed to labor because she was high risk for possible uterine rupture. They told me that the insurance policy she had required trial of labor on all previous Caesarean sections. They should be made accountable for the death of one of my nicest patients. I will testify for the family."

"I would, too. This catastrophe should teach the insurance company a lesson. They are trying to set the trend of medical practice according to how much profit they want to make. It will serve them right, if they get hit for a lot of money, hopefully enough to bankrupt the insurance company."

"Let me talk to John, please. Thank you for calling me and letting me know."

Dr. McKinney handed the phone to John Renly. "Dr. Kelvey wants to talk to you."

"John, I am sorry to hear about Gina. I know how you feel. I am coming down to see you."

"Thank you, Dr. Kelvey. You were right all the way about Gina's fears of going into labor. I will wait for you."

In the meantime, Laura called from the emergency room.

"How did Mrs. Renly do?"

The delivery room nurse started sobbing and said, "She expired twenty minutes ago. She died from too much blood loss. She died of cardiac arrest."

"Oh, my God, this is terrible! I hope the family goes after the insurance company for trying to set the trend of medical practice. The public needs to be educated on how these powerful, greedy, insurance companies manipulate the healthcare system in order to increase their profit. It is about time that someone stands up against such a privileged industry."

"I agree with you, Dr. Secula."

"Thank you for your time."

Laura was exhausted by the time she got up the next morning. She rushed to the cafeteria to get a cup of coffee before she went to Northend Hospital.

As soon as she arrived at Northend Hospital, she heard her name being paged. She went to the information desk.

"Hello, this is Dr. Secula."

"Laura, the basement is done. You can even start moving tonight. Jeanie, Jennifer, and I will be waiting at your apartment. We will make you dinner, too. I know you are very tired. Michael told me that you did not even have a chance to call him."

"I will see you tonight, Mom. Thanks. I cannot talk too much. I will be late for the operating room."

"Bye, Laura."

By the time Laura arrived home from work, Mrs. Secula and Jeanie were already preparing dinner. Michael was playing with Jennifer. Laura kissed her mom and Jeanie. She then joined Michael and Jennifer.

"Jennifer, starting tomorrow, you will see more of your Mommy and Daddy. You will be playing with Daddy everyday. You will have two more people to spoil you."

Jennifer just looked at her mommy and smiled.

After dinner, Mrs. Secula, Jeanie, and Laura started packing all the small stuff which they could put in the trunk of Jeanie's car. They left around ten in the evening.

"Michael, let's sleep. I am exhausted from working at Southern Hospital. There was a maternal death. It was so sad. It was the insurance company's fault. The insurance company carried a clause in its contract with the healthcare insurance of her husband's employer that all previous Caesarean sections should have a trial of labor."

"Then the family should go after his employer, too. That trial of labor clause was put in the contract to save money for the employer and to increase the profit of the insurance company. Each and everyone of them should be accountable for their actions."

"I could not agree more. This profit-motivated healthcare system is the cause of unnecessary deaths and suffering of patients and their families. The public had been and is being victimized by a cruel, unjust healthcare system which is about to collapse and which is under a lot of stress from insoluble social issues and twisted moral values."

"You are right. Probably, it will take decades before the solution to this problem is found."

"It will take a miracle."

"You are right. Time will tell."

On Saturday morning, Laura and Michael woke up very early. The movers came around nine o'clock. By eleven o'clock, the apartment was emptied. Laura and Michael stayed behind so that they could clean the apartment and return the keys to the manager.

By one o'clock, they were on their way to Kalina St.. The mover had already left. Mrs. Secula and Jeanie were busy arranging their things. Jennifer was playing in her playpen. Laura and Michael hugged Jennifer. Jennifer was happy to see her parents. There was a twinkle in her smiling blue eyes.

"Michael, look at Jennifer closely. Everyday she starts to look more and more like you!"

"I know. Probably, we should have named her Michelle."

"No, Jennifer fits her to a 'T'."

"I am just kidding, Laura!"

"I know, but I love the name Jennifer!"

By five o'clock, the basement apartment was completely settled. All that needed to be arranged were the books. Michael could do that on Monday.

Michael and Laura went to St. Archangel's Church. The church was not crowded. No one looked at Michael, for no one would ever suspect that he had AIDS. The only thing wrong with him were his positive HIV and Western Blot tests. Also, he felt weak some days and had occasional lapses of memory, but these were things which were not discernible by any but the most loving eyes.

On Monday morning, Laura left early for work. She turned on the car radio full blast to keep her awake. There was an interruption of the music because of a very important announcement: "After several days of investigation, the Healthcare Financing Administration has decided to suspend the Medicare participation of Southern Hospital indefinitely. The hospital has been fined $50,000.00 for not admitting a 16-year-old girl who later died at Northend Hospital because of hemorrhage. The physician involved will be fined and punished accordingly. The Wobble Abortion Clinic is presently being investigated for possible fraud and homicide. The doctor who did the abortion is being investigated as well."

Laura thought, "It serves them right. They don't care about anything except the bottom line."

Laura and Michael were waiting patiently for the T-cell count. Dr. McIntyre had been on vacation for ten days now. Hopefully, by the time he got back, he would have the result. Michael had left their new number with Dr. McIntyre's secretary. It was now the thirteenth day since the blood test was drawn. Michael even tried calling the university, but the report was not in yet. The waiting made Michael fidgety. He paced the house all the time. Jennifer kept him busy, though. Every morning he took Jennifer to the patio with him and showed her pictures of birds, animals, and flowers. Sometimes, he tried to talk to her in her own, sweet little way.

He could even sense when Jennifer's diapers were wet. Michael was a doting, loving father.

On the fifteenth day after the blood test was drawn, Dr. McIntyre called Michael.

"Michael, I have to see you and Laura in the office. Please, try to come as soon as possible. I want to increase your AZT to one thousand mg per day, too. Please call me back after you talk to Laura."

Michael was stunned. He started sobbing. He called Laura immediately.

"Laura, do you have time to come home now and take me to Dr. McIntyre's office?"

"Of course I do, and, even if I didn't, somebody would just have to cover for me. Michael, I know it is bad news. I can tell by the tone of your voice. I will be home shortly."

As soon as Laura arrived home, she saw Michael sitting in front of the study desk.

Michael's tear-streaked face had been ravaged by sadness.

Laura hugged Michael. They both started crying.

"We have to practice what we preach to our patients. We have to hope and pray that we will have the faith, courage, and strength to deal with our problems. I know it is not easy. But we will be able to handle it because we have each other. We have a supportive family and loving friends. We have it better than other people with AIDS. Some don't even have families and friends who care about them. Some of them just sadly and painfully lie in bed without any hope or reassurance from anyone. They are just waiting to die! Michael, your illness brought more positive things into our lives. It has strengthened our love for each other. It has not diminished our identities, but instead has enhanced our relationship and commitment to each other."

"Thank you for your pep talk, Laura."

"This is not pep talk, Michael. This is reality and truth. Michael, let's go. We will talk to Mom and Jeanie as soon as we get back. Did you get something to eat, Michael?"

"Yes, I did. But I was not really that hungry. Mom and Jennifer walked to the supermarket. We will just call them when we get to Dr. McIntyre's office."

Laura drove very fast. They got to the Center City office of Dr. McIntyre in no time.

As soon as they arrived, the receptionist ushered them in to Dr. McIntyre's consultation room.

"How are you, both?", asked Dr. McIntyre, while shaking Michael's and then Laura's hand. "Please, take your seats."

"Dr. McIntyre, what did my T-cell count show?"

"Michael, I have to be truthful. Your T-cells are down to 380 per cubic mm. The peripheral blood smear also showed macrocytic anemia and folic acid deficiency which is to be expected with AZT therapy due to the bone marrow toxicity. I will have to examine you now and see if you have developed some other symptoms which you might have completely ignored."

"The other symptoms which I have noticed are muscle aches, occasional forgetfulness, and tiredness, especially in the afternoons."

"Well, myalgia and being tired are expected symptoms. I want to send you to a neurologist to see if your forgetfulness has any relation to AIDS. Dr. Sampler has an office across the street. I am going to call his office now to see if he can squeeze you into his schedule today."

Dr. McIntyre called Dr. Sampler.

"Sure, I can see Dr. Olsire in an hour. I will tell my secretary to call your office as soon as we are ready for him."

"Thank you, Dr. Sampler."

Michael and Dr. McIntyre went back to the consultation room where Laura was waiting.

"Michael, I have to increase your AZT as I have said. I have to put you on iron and folic acid, too. Laura, do you have any questions?"

"No, Dr. McIntyre. I just want you to know that we appreciate your kindness and concern for Michael."

"Michael, you can start the extra dose of AZT now. I have some extra capsules here."

"Thank you, Dr. McIntyre."

"I will wait for you here. Please come back after you see Dr. Sampler. I want to know what his opinion is."

"We will be back, Dr. McIntyre."

Dr. Sampler's secretary directed them to his consultation room as soon as they arrived.

Dr. Sampler took Michael's history while Laura listened.

"Have you noticed any lapses in your memory, Michael?"

"Yes, I have. It started more than eight weeks ago."

"Did you have diplopia (seeing double), blurring of vision, or headaches?"

"No."

"Well, Michael, I will have to see you at least twice a month just to monitor you closely and to see if your forgetfulness is related to AIDS. Dr. McIntyre is waiting for you in his office. I will give him a call."

Dr. McIntyre was on the phone with Dr. Sampler when they arrived in his office. He shook their hands as soon as he hung up the phone.

"I have good news for both of you. Dr. Sampler cannot make any definite conclusion about Michael's memory lapses. He will see you in two weeks. Please drop by my office after he sees you then. Here are some more AZT capsules for you."

"Thank you, Dr. McIntyre."

"If you have any questions, please feel free to call me."

"Thank you for the samples, Dr. McIntyre."

"I will see you in two weeks."

Michael and Laura had forgotten to call Mrs. Secula while they were at Dr. McIntyre's office. Mrs. Secula had been looking for Michael. She had called Laura at Northend Hospital. The surgical resident had informed her that Laura had left the hospital to take Michael to the doctor. Mrs. Secula had been relieved upon hearing that. She then decided to put Jennifer to sleep so she could cook.

Laura and Michael reached home in no time. They were barely inside their basement apartment when the phone rang. It was Dr. Simmons.

"Michael, we are scheduled to have the deposition in ten days. I told Mr. Edward Sanborne to talk to Mr. Smith about deposing all of us at the same time. He said that it might take a whole day. I have to call James Dillon and John Miller so they can fly in for the deposition."

"Dr. Simmons, please tell Mr. Sanborne to ask Mr. Smith that we be deposed at the Secula residence. The patio will accommodate all of us. I just came from Drs. McIntyre and Sampler. My T-cell count is down to 380 per cubic mm. This is the reason I want the deposition here. I don't know in what physical condition I will be in ten days."

"I understand, Michael. Please call me if you need anything."

"Thank you, Dr. Simmons. Let me know what Sanborne and Smith think about my idea."

"I will call you in a couple of days, Michael."

"I will be waiting for your call, Dr. Simmons. Give our 'hello' to Debbie. She is really doing a good job."

"I will."

"Laura, I think we better call Father John tonight. I am afraid my illness is taking a shorter course than I expected."

"Whatever you say, Michael. We have to tell Mom and Jeanie tonight, too. Let's go up and have lunch before I go back to work. I think Jennifer is sleeping. Our poor baby, if she only knew what was going on in our lives, it would break her young heart."

"It is better that she does not realize what is going on. She can just go on with her sweet angelic ways."

"I agree with you."

Mrs. Secula was setting the table when Michael and Laura came up.

"Lunch will be ready shortly. How was your testing, Michael?"

"It was not that great, Mom. But we will all survive this ordeal. Dr. McIntyre sent me to a neurologist, Dr. Sampler, to check for neurological manifestations. So far, he is not sure. Dr. McIntyre increased the dose of my AZT and gave me folic acid and iron. I have to go back to both doctors in two weeks. They were both optimistic. Dr. McIntyre gave me my supply of AZT for one month. That will help us save money."

"Michael, thank you for all your optimism. It makes things easier for all the people who love you."

CHAPTER XXXI

Laura was getting ready to go to work when the phone rang. It was James Dillon. He had just arrived last night from Dublin, Ireland.

"Hello, Laura. May I speak to Michael, please? How have you been?"

"Well, Dr. Simmons must have told you about Michael."

"Yes, he did. I was very upset when I received the bad news. How is Michael doing now?"

"We just got the bad news six days ago. But we are dealing with it very well. Michael's T-cells are now down to 380 per cubic mm. His AZT was increased to 1,000 mg. He was also put on iron and folic acid. I am going to wake him up so that you can talk to him. Hold on."

Laura went into the bedroom where Michael was sleeping.

"Michael, Michael, please wake up. James Dillon is on the phone."

"Who?"

"James Dillon is on the phone. I have to go to work now. He is on the phone. Breakfast is on the table. See you tonight."

Michael slowly walked towards the study desk.

"James, how are you? When did you arrive?"

"I arrived last night from Dublin. I am staying with Dr. Simmons. We are expecting Ann and John Miller tomorrow. We will visit you and get together with you before our deposition."

"Is Mr. Sanborne coming, too?"

"I don't think so. We really don't have much to discuss. This case is just a waste of our time."

"Dr. Simmons has a copy of Patty Singleton's transcribed deposition. Did he show it to you?"

"No, I think he will bring it when we come and visit you."

"I think that is a good idea."

"So, how are you doing, Michael?"

"Not so good. Dr. McIntyre had increased my AZT to 1,000 mg. I hope I don't develop the more toxic reactions in addition to my anemia."

"I hope so, too. I have to get some sleep. Dr. Simmons is still asleep. We will call you back as soon as John Miller arrives. Get some rest, Michael. Bye."

"Thanks for calling, James."

Michael went back to sleep. He felt so rundown. By ten in the morning, Mrs. Secula came down with Jennifer to see how Michael was doing. Michael's face looked anguished and pale. Mrs. Secula was in tears as she observed Michael's facial expression. At seeing Michael, Jennifer squealed in delight which awakened him.

"Mom, I am sorry. I did not realize that you and Jennifer had been watching me in my sleep. I feel very tired today. I was just talking to James Dillon a while ago."

"How is Dr. Dillon?"

"He is fine. They will be coming down here in two days before our deposition so that we can study the chart of Charlie Singleton and read Patty's deposition."

"You can tell them that they can stay for dinner."

"Thanks, Mom. I will do that."

Michael took Jennifer from Mrs. Secula, and they all went upstairs for breakfast.

"I bathed Jennifer while we were waiting for you to wake up."

"Thanks, Mom."

Michael sat Jennifer in her high chair and gave her milk and some baby food.

"We have not called Father John yet about the report of my new laboratory testing. We just have to let him know tonight. I have to remind Laura when she gets home."

Ring===Ring===Ring

Michael picked up the phone. It was Dr. Simmons.

"Michael, I just talked to Mr. Sanborne. Robert Smith has agreed to depose all of us at the same time at your place. It will take the whole day. Mr. Sanborne is coming to discuss the case with us, too."

"That would be fine. I don't care if the deposition lasts more than a day as long as it is held at Kalina St.."

"How are you feeling, Michael?"

"Just tired, Dr. Simmons. Dr. McIntyre has been very accommodating. I will see him again in two weeks. He even personally called Dr. Sampler to see me the same day that Laura and I were in his office for adjustment of my AZT. He is a very nice man. A caring doctor."

"That is why I referred you to him. I knew you would like him. How is Laura holding up?"

"She is doing good. But I am not sure she has really accepted my illness or realized that one day I will just be gone suddenly."

"You cannot blame her. But at least her work keeps her occupied."

"I know. How is Debbie?"

"Debbie is doing good. She just loves her work."

"I am glad for her. I hope she is not working too hard. When will John Miller be coming?"

"I think tomorrow. Please, give Laura my best. Jennifer must be getting big now."

"She is. She keeps her grandmom active and busy."

"Michael, we will be seeing you on Wednesday. Does ten o'clock in the morning sound good to you?"

"That would be fine, Dr. Simmons. I will see you all then."

"Bye, Michael."

Michael went down to the basement to call up his AIDS buddies. He usually did these phone interviews from eleven o'clock in the morning until three in the afternoon. Most of his buddies lived in apartments, but none of their neighbors knew that they were afflicted with AIDS. Some of them lived in houses run by volunteers. The addresses of these houses were kept secret for fear of reprisal or intimidation from an uneducated, narrow-minded public. Michael's phone calls had meant so much emotionally to his fellow AIDS victims. He wished he could do more for them.

Michael did not eat lunch until three o'clock in the afternoon. Laura came home late because there had been several shooting victims brought to the trauma center. She had to assist the cardiovascular surgeon in a thoracic exploration. Four people had died in the shooting spree. The police were still investigating the incident when she had left for home.

"Michael, how was your day?"

"I talked to Dr. Simmons today. Robert Smith agreed to have the deposition here."

"I have to take off that day."

"Why?"

"I have to see if this guy is the same Robert Smith Charlie used to talk about."

"How will you know?"

"I don't know. I just have to observe him."

"Laura, you cannot be included in the deposition. You will have to stay inside the basement apartment and watch from inside."

"I know."

"We have to call Father John tonight. We forgot to call him six days ago."

"Let's go downstairs. I will check first if Jennifer is still sleeping."

Laura went inside Jennifer's room. Little Jennifer was sleeping peacefully.

"Come on, Michael, let's call Father John."

Michael dialed Father John's telephone number, but it was busy.

"We will try after ten o'clock."

Mrs. Secula came down to talk to Michael and Laura.

"Mom, I did not realize you were still awake."

"I have to wait for Jeanie. She attended a retirement party. She will not be home until twelve tonight."

"Mom, I forgot to tell you that our lawyer is coming, too, on Wednesday."

"That will be fine with me, Michael."

"I will be here, too, Mom."

"I was sure you would be, Laura."

Michael tried to call Father John again. Finally, Father John answered.

"Father, this is Michael. How are you? How is your fund-raising coming along?"

"We are doing fine. We are about to reach our campaign goal."

"That's marvelous. Father, I just want to give you an update of my medical condition. My T-cells are down. I am now on a higher dose of AZT. I hope it helps."

"Michael, what can I say except trust God's wisdom. Everything happens for a reason. I am sure Laura is coping very well."

"She is. I am very proud of her. She is a gem."

Let me talk to her."

"Hello, Father John. When are you going to come for a visit?"

"As soon as I finish this fund-raising campaign. Laura, I just want to thank you and your family for your unwavering love and support for Michael."

"Father, this is what marriage is all about. If only people could truly understand and analyze what the marriage vow is, there would be less divorce."

"I cannot agree more. How is Jennifer?"

"Jennifer is sleeping upstairs. She is growing and getting bigger every day. Father, we will be expecting you soon then. Do you want to talk to Michael again?"

"I think we have talked enough. Just tell him I will come for a visit as soon as I can. Good night, Laura."

"Good night, Father."

Two days later, Drs. Simmons, John Miller, James Dillon, and Michael were discussing with Mr. Sanborne about Charlie Singleton's illness. Mr. Sanborne decided that Dr. Simmons was only peripherally involved since he did not talk to or examine Charlie. The main defendants were Michael, James Dillon, and John Miller. He told them that he would try to get Dr. Simmons dismissed as a defendant. The doctors went over Charlie's medical and surgical history from the day of admission to the two emergency operations he had had. Their defense was that blood was given in an emergency situation, and, at that time, that there was no sophisticated laboratory testing to detect the presence of AIDS. They all agreed that the best way to prevent Mr. Robert Smith from playing them against each other was for them to be deposed at the same time. Since Dr. Simmons' involvement was actually nil, Mr. Sanborne had suggested to the insurance company that he be represented by another law firm. The medical liability insurance company, however, had decided against Mr. Sanborne's suggestion in order to save more money. The four doctors also tried to update Mr. Sanborne about the epidemiology of AIDS, the current concepts, its complications, and treatment.

"This will be the first AIDS case that will go on trial in Philadelphia. I think Robert Smith presumes that he will set a precedent in this case."

"That remains to be seen. He will have to have an expert to do that. AIDS as a disease is complex. The virus keeps on multiplying every second; it will be extremely hard for scientists to find the cure."

"I couldn't agree more."

"Mr. Sanborne, I must tell you something confidential. I don't know if it will help our case. I myself have developed AIDS from Charlie. John Miller accidentally dropped on my hand the knife I used during Charlie's second emergency surgery. I don't even know if I will still be around during the trial. But, I think you should put that on the record. The truth should be told. Charlie's AIDS was not caused by blood transfusion but by drug addiction."

"I see. Thank you for telling me. Is there any other information that we should discuss about this case?"

"How about the hepatitis? Shouldn't we clarify it, too?" asked John Miller.

"Well, there was really no available test at the time of Charlie's illness to test for hepatitis C. So, we cannot just blame it on the blood transfusion. All his blood testing at that time was positive for hepatitis probably due to contaminated needles during cocaine injections by, according to Charlie, a certain hot-shot lawyer named Robert Smith."

"What? Robert Smith was giving cocaine injections?"

"We don't really know who Robert Smith, the drug dealer, is. There are about twenty lawyers in Philadelphia whose name is Robert Smith. We have to do further investigation about this Robert Smith. If we get evidence against him as being a drug dealer, then we can turn the table against him. That would also be the end of his legal career."

"It could not happen to a worse man."

"Have you read Mrs. Patricia Singleton's deposition?"

"Yes, and we feel there is really nothing derogatory in her deposition. In fact, her deposition is very complimentary to Michael."

"I think so, too."

"Well, since we have nothing more to talk about, I will be seeing all of you here with Robert Smith in a few days."

"We will see you then."

"Michael, we better let you rest. You look exhausted," said Dr. Simmons.

On Friday, September 15, 1985, Michael had a chance to see first hand how the legal process operated. This was also the first time for Dr. Simmons, James Dillon, and John Miller to see how an eminent medico-legal malpractice lawyer operated and manipulated the legal process. Laura helped Michael put on his business suit.

Robert Smith and the court reporter arrived promptly. The deposition started at ten in the morning.

The first doctor to be deposed was Dr. Simmons:

"Do you remember Mr. Charlie Singleton?"

"No."

"How many times did you see this patient?"

"Once."

"Did you have any doctor-patient relationship?"

"No."

In what capacity did you see him?"

"As a bystander."

"What do you mean?"

"I saw the patient while Dr. James Dillon was examining him in the accident ward. I was waiting for Dr. James Dillon to finish his physical examination and his conversation with Dr. Michael Olsire."

"Did you participate in the care of this patient?"

"No."

"According to the answer to the interrogatories sent by you, you were a professor at the University. How long had you been teaching?"

"Yes, I was a professor. I taught for forty years."

"Are you an author, too?"

"Yes, I am."

"That means that all you know about medicine is through book learning without practical experience?"

"It is the other way around. I write about my practical experience."

"How many cases of AIDS have you seen?"

"I don't remember the exact number."

"That will be all, Dr. Simmons. I would like to depose Dr. James Dillon next."

"Where are you practicing now?"

"In Dublin, Ireland."

"Do you practice full-time?"

"Part-time."

"Do you teach at a university?"

"Yes."

"Where?"

"Trinity University."

"In what capacity?"

"I am an instructor in surgery."

"Did you know Charlie Singleton?"

"Yes."

"Did you take care of him?"

"Yes."

"Did you have a doctor-patient relationship?"

"I thought so."

"Did you do the first operation on Charlie Singleton?"

"Yes, I did."

"Did you transfuse him?"

"Yes."

"Why?"

"That was the only recourse left to save his life."

"Did you explain to him the risks of blood transfusion such as AIDS, hepatitis, and renal shutdown?"

"No, he would not have understood any explanation."

"Why?"

"He was spaced out."

"Was someone with him at that time?"

"Nobody was with him."

"Who took care of him post-operatively?"

"Dr. Olsire and I."

"Do you think Dr. Olsire did his post-operative care follow-up well?"

"Absolutely."

"Were you in the hospital when Charlie Singleton was readmitted with his intestines hanging out (dehiscence) from his abdomen?"

"No."

"Who took care of him that night?"

"Dr. Michael Olsire."

"Don't you think something is wrong with your surgical technique when a patient comes back to the accident ward with an opened incision and bowels hanging out from the incision?"

"No."

"How do you explain Mr. Singleton's dehiscence after his discharge?"

"Mr. Singleton was not discharged. He left the hospital without medical advice. I don't know what he did after he left the hospital."

"Did you try to locate him after he disappeared from his room?"

"Yes."

"Were you successful in locating him?"

"No."

"How did he get back to the hospital?"

"By rescue squad."

"Who took care of him and fixed the dehiscence?"

"Dr. Michael Olsire."

"Who scrubbed with Dr. Olsire?"

"Dr. John Miller."

"That will be all. I have to depose Dr. John Miller next. Where are you practicing now?"

"I am practicing in Ohio."

"What specialty?"

"General surgery."

"Do you teach in a medical school, too?"

"No."

"Do you plan to teach in a medical school?"

"No, I plan to do full-time private practice."

"Where did you finish your residency?"

"At University Hospital."

"Did you take any fellowship?"

"No."

"How many cases of AIDS had you seen during your residency?"

"I can't remember the exact number."

"Can you guess?"

"No."

"Did you take care of Mr. Charlie Singleton?"

"Not exactly."

"Did you assist in any of his operations?"

"Yes, the second operation."

"What do you mean by 'second operation'?"

"The closure of the abdominal incision following dehiscence."

"Was he tested for AIDS with this admission?"

"Yes."

"Are you sure?"

"I am absolutely positive."

"What was the result of the test?"

"It was negative."

"Does blood transfusion expose one to risk of AIDS and hepatitis?"

"Yes."

"Do you think Mr. Charlie's Singleton's AIDS and hepatitis were caused by blood transfusion?"

"No."

"Are you sure?"

"Yes."

"What makes you so sure?"

"Charlie Singleton had been involved in using and selling drugs in Center City. He had been a drug abuser for at least two years before his admission to the hospital."

Robert Smith was stunned when John Miller said that. He looked pale for a few seconds but immediately bounced back.

"I want to depose Dr. Michael Olsire now. How many years of surgical residency have you had?"

"Five years."

"Did you take any fellowship?"

"Yes."

"How many years?"

"Two years."

"Do you remember Charlie Singleton?"

"Hardly."

"Did you take care of him?"

"Yes."

"How long did you take care of him?"

"I don't remember."

"Did you operate on him?"

"I think so."

"Did you have a doctor-patient relationship?"

"I don't know."

"Why is it you don't remember anything? From all the deposed doctors' accounts, you were really close to Charlie Singleton."

"I am really not sure. I am not feeling very well."

Robert Smith was getting annoyed at Michael for answering his interrogations that way.

"Dr. Olsire, please answer my questions truthfully to the best of your knowledge. If you don't answer me now, I can get those answers at the trial. How many times did you operate on Charlie Singleton?"

"I don't remember."

"Dr. Olsire, I am sick and tired of your answers! I am terminating this deposition right now! I will see you all in court!"

Robert Smith left in a huff without saying a word. Mr. Sanborne stayed for a few minutes.

"Don't worry about Robert Smith's tantrums. He does this all the time to intimidate the witnesses into answering all his questions. Don't let him get to you. Have a nice day."

CHAPTER XXXII

Laura was misty-eyed as she looked through the patio window. From the little conversation she had overheard, she knew that Robert Smith left hurriedly because Michael was not able to answer his interrogations. She perceived that Michael's memory loss was something very serious. She tried to camouflage her feelings as she went out to the patio where the four doctors were conferring about the temperamental and arrogant behavior of Robert Smith. Laura broke into the conversation.

"How did you make out with your deposition?"

"We thought we did fairly well. Michael did well by deliberately forgetting everything about Charlie Singleton. Michael's answers so annoyed Robert Smith that he cut short Michael's deposition."

Laura bit her tongue. She knew Michael's memory lapse was not deliberate. Many morbid suppositions about Michael's illness were running through her mind. "Does Michael have lymphoma of the brain secondary to AIDS? Does Michael have a brain tumor independent of AIDS? Is Michael at the terminal stage of AIDS?"

"Laura, you are in deep thought."

"I am sorry, Dr. Simmons. I am thinking about something very important. It is already five o'clock. Why don't you stay for dinner?"

"Laura, we appreciate your invitation, but we promised Debbie that we would take her out to dinner tonight. We will have to pick up Debbie at her office."

"Please say 'hi' to her for us."

"We will do that."

"I will call you before I leave for Ireland."

"Take care, Michael. Goodbye."

"Goodbye, everyone."

Laura and Michael went upstairs to have dinner with Mrs. Secula, Jeanie, and Jennifer. Michael was very quiet. He did not talk much at the dinner table. Laura was very disturbed. She decided that she should talk to Michael after dinner. She could feel that Michael was in pain. He seemed a little depressed. Laura could sense that Michael was trying to keep his suffering to himself. "Is Michael trying to spare me pain?"

"Michael, let's go down the basement after Jeanie and I finish washing the dishes. We have to talk."

"No problem. I will tuck Jennifer in bed while you and Jeanie are washing dishes. Jennifer looks tired and sleepy."

"It will not take long for me and Jeanie to clean up. By the time Jennifer falls asleep, we will be finished cleaning the whole kitchen."

Michael took Jennifer to her room. Jennifer started crying.

"Laura, please get me a diaper for Jennifer. She is wet."

"I will be there shortly."

Laura took the diaper to Jennifer's room and gave it to Michael. Laura looked at Michael closely. There was so much sadness in his eyes.

"Michael, how are you feeling?"

"I feel fine."

"I don't think you really feel fine. Please tell me what is bothering you. You look so sad. You look like someone who has just lost his whole world."

"Laura, we will talk about this later. As soon as Jennifer falls asleep, we will talk downstairs."

"Is that a deal?"

"Yes, it is a deal."

By the time Laura got out of Jennifer's room, Jeanie was done with the dishes. Later, after Jennifer had fallen asleep, Laura and Michael went down to the basement to talk.

"Michael, please level with me. I know you don't feel right. I've noticed the hesitation when you walk. You have hard time remembering things, too. Do you also have double vision?"

"I do, Laura."

"Why didn't you tell me? When did you start having all these symptoms?"

"Two days ago. You were very tired from working, and you have not had enough sleep for the past three days so I decided to wait before I told you."

"Michael, please don't worry about me. I can handle it. I am going to call Dr. McIntyre tomorrow to see if he can squeeze you into his schedule. We are also going to see Dr. Sampler. I hope Dr. Sampler orders a CAT Scan on you. Michael, I am so afraid. I don't know what to say."

"Laura, I understand all your fears, but we just have to accept God's will."

Laura hugged Michael. She could not control herself anymore. She started crying.

"Michael, you must understand why I am crying. I am crying to be able to cope with our problem. This is my only outlet. I don't want to get depressed. I just want to cry my heart out. Even my soul is being tried. And, my heart is aching."

Michael stroked Laura's hair.

"Laura, it is alright for you to cry. I understand."

"I think we better go to sleep so that we will wake up early. I am not going to work tomorrow. I have already called our chief resident."

Laura was awake by six o'clock. She went upstairs to cook breakfast for everyone. Mrs. Secula and Jennifer were still asleep. As soon as breakfast was ready, Laura woke up Michael. Jennifer, Jeanie, and Mrs. Secula were awake by seven o'clock. Everyone had a hearty breakfast. Jeanie left for work at eight o'clock.

"Mom, Michael and I are going to see Dr. McIntyre today. I am not going to work today. I called my senior resident last night."

Jennifer was still yawning and quite cranky when Laura took her from Mrs. Secula.

"Jennifer, Daddy and Mommy are going downtown so Daddy can have his regular check-up."

Laura was misty-eyed while trying to talk to Jennifer.

At eight-thirty, Michael and Laura went down to the basement. Laura called Dr. McIntyre's office. The phone was busy. It took her thirty minutes to get through on the phone. Dr. McIntyre's secretary squeezed them in for an eleven o'clock appointment.

The drive to Center City was quite hectic. Laura had to go around several blocks before she could find a parking space. Dr. McIntyre's office was crowded when they arrived. Apparently, Dr. McIntyre had had to leave for an emergency call in the hospital. The patients ahead of Laura and Michael were waiting patiently. Laura asked the secretary of Dr. McIntyre to call Dr. Sampler's office. Laura had tried to call Dr. Sampler's office before they had left for Center City, but had been unable to get through.

"Dr. Secula, Dr. Sampler is on the line now."

"Thank you. Dr. Sampler, this is Laura Secula-Olsire. I would like to know if you have an opening in your office schedule for this afternoon. Dr. McIntyre has been called to the hospital. He has not seen the five patients who came ahead of us, so probably he will not be able to see Michael until this afternoon."

"Would you be able to come to my office now?"

"I think so."

"Well, then I can see Michael right away. I will be finished talking with my last patient by the time you get here."

"Thank you very much, Dr. Sampler."

"You are welcome, Dr. Secula."

As soon as Laura and Michael arrived at Dr. Sampler's office, they were ushered by his secretary into his consultation room.

"How are you, Michael?"

"I don't feel that great, Dr. Sampler. I have been having lapses of memory, weakness, fatigue, and occasional double vision."

"Let me examine you. Laura, you can join us in the examining room if you want."

Laura followed them to the examining room. Dr. Sampler did a complete neurological examination on Michael.

"Michael, you will have to get a CAT Scan of the brain as soon as possible. I will call the X-Ray department now. I will see if they can squeeze you into tomorrow's schedule."

"Thank you, Dr. Sampler."

Dr. Sampler called the X-Ray department of the university hospital. He was able to get an appointment for Michael for ten-thirty the next morning. Laura and Michael thanked Dr. Sampler and left for Dr. McIntyre's office. By the time they got back to Dr. McIntyre's office, there was only one patient left in the waiting room.

Dr. McIntyre took them to his office immediately and talked to both of them. Laura and Michael were both very attentive of what Dr. McIntyre was saying.

"Michael, you have to go for another T-cell count tomorrow. We have to know how you are responding to the increased dosage of AZT."

"Well, I will be killing two birds at a time then. Dr. Sampler has scheduled me for a CAT Scan, too. We will be in the hospital for half a day probably."

"No problem, Michael. I will drive you there tomorrow."

"But, Laura, you have to go to work."

"I have decided to take a leave of absence. I am going to take care of you myself."

"But I can still take care of myself."

"I know, but you don't only need physical care. You also need emotional and spiritual care. Michael, please, I want to do this for myself, too. I do not want to be an 'if' person."

"Whatever you want to do, Laura."

"Thank you, Michael. I am going to take you home. Afterwards, I will get some of my stuff at Northend Hospital. I will also have to talk to the senior resident and the chief of surgery."

Dr. McIntyre just stood there, listening and watching the interaction between Laura and Michael. He could not help but admire their love and respect for each other. He said to himself, "I wish they had more time left to spend together." He was misty-eyed as he watched Laura and Michael leave.

It was almost five o'clock by the time they arrived home. Laura called the senior resident and told him that she was taking an indefinite leave of absence. The senior resident said he would relay the message to the Chief of Surgery. Laura had to talk to the Chief of Surgery personally and had to submit a letter for a leave of absence request.

"I cannot go there tomorrow to talk to the chief. I will have to do it on Thursday."

"That will be fine with me."

Michael, Laura, Mrs. Secula, and Jennifer had dinner. After dinner, Michael took Jennifer to the basement and played with her. Laura and Mrs. Secula were washing the dishes when Laura started sobbing.

"Laura, what's wrong?"

"Mom, I did not hear any good news about Michael today. Michael's condition is getting worse."

"In what way?"

"He has some nervous system involvement. He is going to have a repeat blood test and a CAT Scan of the brain tomorrow. I am going to take a leave of absence indefinitely. Michael is terminally ill."

"Laura, I understand what you are feeling right now. But the only shield we have in the wake of an impending tragedy is our Faith and God's grace. Death is a divine plan. We can postpone it, but we cannot prevent it. God put us on earth for a reason and for a certain time. It is He who decides when He wants us back in His kingdom."

"I know, Mom, but I have not really accepted the fact that in such a short span of time, I will be losing Michael. And Jennifer will lose her Daddy! She cannot even understand what is going on in our lives. She will never remember what a loving father Michael was."

"Laura, I think Jennifer can sense that Michael might not be here for long. Sometimes, Jennifer looks at Michael and smiles, and then looks back at him and cries. Even a baby growing inside a mother's womb feels the stresses and tensions of his mother; much more can a little girl of Jennifer's age feel."

"I agree with you, Mom. But it is quite difficult for me to comprehend all the things which are evolving so fast."

Laura, wipe your eyes. I think Michael is coming up."

"Laura, I want to call Father John and talk to him."

"Michael, I will be down as soon as we finish washing dishes."

Mrs. Secula and Laura went down together. Mrs. Secula took Jennifer with her upstairs.

Michael dialed Father John's number.

"Hello, Father John. This is Michael. How are you?"

"I am doing fine. How about you, Michael? How are you doing with your treatment?"

"Not too well, Father John. I have developed some neurological symptoms. I am going to have my blood testing repeated and a CAT Scan. Laura wants to talk to you."

"Hello, Father John."

"Laura, how are you doing?"

"Not too good, Father John. I think you should come down and visit us as soon as possible."

"Do you think that Michael is really that sick?"

"Yes, Father John. I cannot really talk now. Please come soon."

"I will be there as soon as I can. I will call you back as soon as I have made arrangements for my flight."

"We will be seeing you soon, Father John. Good night."

"Good night, Laura."

Laura and Michael woke up early the next day. Laura cooked a hot breakfast for Michael. Jennifer and Mrs. Secula were still asleep when Michael and Laura left.

The drive to the University took an hour because of the early morning traffic. They had a hard time finding a parking space. Finally, they found one at a nearby restaurant.

"Laura, I feel very weak. I don't think I can make it to the laboratory. I can hardly see. I am not only having double vision. I think I've lost my vision."

"Michael, please don't talk like that!"

"I am not kidding, Laura. I cannot see!"

"You wait here, Michael. I am going to lock all the doors. I am going to make a phone call."

Laura went to the phone booth in the hospital lobby. She called Dr. Simmons at his home.

"Hello, Dr. Simmons," sobbed Laura.

"What's the matter, Laura? You sound so distressed. Where are you? Is Michael with you, too?"

"Yes, Dr. Simmons. Michael is with me. He is supposed to get a CAT Scan today, but, all of a sudden, he lost his vision."

"What?"

"Yes, Michael cannot see! He is waiting for me in the car."

"Call Debbie at work so she can come and help you with Michael. I will be there as soon as possible."

"Thank you, Dr. Simmons."

Laura called Debbie at work.

"Debbie, Michael and I are near the University in a parking lot between two restaurants. Michael just completely lost his vision. I hope you can come and help me get him out of the car."

"I will be there as soon as I can, Laura."

In fifteen minutes, Debbie arrived at the parking lot. She appeared very upset. She could not believe that this was the same handsome Michael who used to come to her house for dinner every now and then. He still looked handsome, but was so pale and tired.

"Michael, how are you?"

"Not so good, Debbie. Everything is happening so fast. I am supposed to have a repeat blood count and a CAT Scan today."

"You wait here. I am going to get a wheelchair from the accident ward. We can probably wheel you to the laboratory and the X-Ray department."

"Thank you, Debbie."

"Laura, stay with Michael. Father should be arriving anytime now."

Before Debbie came back with the wheelchair, Dr. Simmons was already in the parking lot looking for Laura's car.

"Dr. Simmons, Dr. Simmons! Michael and I are here."

Finally, Dr. Simmons heard Laura and located her.

"I'm here, Laura."

Laura opened the passenger door so that Dr. Simmons could talk to Michael.

"Michael, how are you? How do you feel?"

"Dr. Simmons, I cannot see!"

"Well, we will just wait for Debbie and then we will take you to the laboratory and X-Ray. I am going to get Dr. Aldrich to check your eyes. We want to know what is going on with you."

"Dr. Simmons, this just happened as soon as Laura parked the car. I was trying to get out of the car, when, all of a sudden, I could not see! As if a flash of lightning had hit my eye! I am very concerned. I am afraid AIDS has affected my brain."

"Michael, please don't draw any rash conclusions until Dr. Aldrich has checked you."

"I understand, Dr. Simmons."

Debbie finally arrived with the wheelchair. Dr. Simmons and Laura helped Michael get out of the car. They went to the laboratory first. Dr. Tearcell was already there when they arrived. He drew Michael's blood and sent it out STAT. Dr. Simmons and Laura wheeled Michael to the X-Ray department. The CAT Scan of the brain was done with the use of contrast medium. The CAT Scan did not show any definite abnormality except for a decreased density of the brain. Dr. Simmons had already made an appointment for Michael with Dr. Aldrich. Dr. Simmons and Laura wheeled Michael to Dr. Aldrich's office. They were ushered in immediately. Upon seeing them, Dr. Aldrich stood up and shook everybody's hands. He did a complete eye examination on Michael.

"Michael, did you have any headache or blurring of vision before you completely lost your vision?"

"Yes, I did, but it was on and off. I just completely ignored the symptoms."

"When did you start having them?"

"Three weeks ago."

"Do you have a headache now?"

"Yes, I do."

"Did you have any fever at all in the past in addition to the headache and blurring of vision which you have experienced?"

"No."

"Michael, your skin feels very warm to me. I will take your temperature."

Three minutes later, Dr. Aldrich took the thermometer from underneath Michael's tongue.

"Michael, your temperature is 102°. You have to be admitted. Your eye examination showed papilledema (increase intracranial pressure), I will call Dr. Sampler and tell him that I am admitting you under his service."

Dr. Aldrich took Laura aside.

"Laura, I think Michael has meningitis. He will need a lumbar tap. The CAT Scan report is not conclusive. I am sorry to give you the bad news."

"I knew it was something like that. I just have difficulty accepting it. I know, too, that this is fatal, and that the clinical course is very stormy. Michael and I have talked about this as a possible complication of AIDS. He does not want to be resuscitated. After the diagnosis is made, I want to take him home. He does not want to die in the hospital. He wants to die in peace at home, cared for by his loved ones."

"I understand, Laura. But he will need constant care."

"I will do that. I have already requested a leave of absence. Excuse me, Dr. Aldrich, I have to call Father John and my Mom and the Director of Surgery at Northend Hospital."

Laura made several phone calls. She did not get Father John. She called her mother and gave her an update of what was going on with Michael. Mrs. Secula said she would keep calling Father John until she got him. She had to call Jeanie at work and tell her about what was going on with Michael. Jeanie and Mrs. Secula would pick up Father John at the airport as soon as they found out the time of his arrival.

Laura called the Director of Surgery at Northend Hospital. She explained to him about Michael's illness.

"You mean to say your husband is terminally ill with AIDS? How come you never told me?"

"I had no reason to tell you."

"But you take care of patients! You are exposing them to AIDS!"

"Dr. Scoop, how narrow-minded and callous can you be! I have no AIDS. I have been tested several times. All my HIV and Western Blot tests came back negative. The last test was done last month."

"Regardless, I will have to insist that you get a complete physical examination and HIV testings before you come back to work."

"I know that and that is exactly what I am planning to do before I come back to work. I know my duties and obligations to my patients. I will never expose any patient unnecessarily to AIDS. Goodbye, Dr. Scoop."

Dr. Scoop was flabbergasted. "This Laura Secula has a mind of her own."

By the time Laura returned to Michael's room, Dr. Sampler had already finished the lumbar tap.

"Laura, I did not wait for you before I did the lumbar tap. I did not want to waste time."

"I can understand, Dr. Sampler."

"The spinal fluid was cloudy. I requested a smear with Indian Ink, chemistry, and microscopic examinations of the spinal fluid."

"How long will it take before we find out?"

"We will find out this afternoon. I will let you know."

By three o'clock, the result of the Indian Ink smear came back as encapsulated yeast. Dr. Sampler came back to Michael's room. Dr. Simmons had been with Laura throughout the ordeal. Debbie had to go back to work. She had been on the phone a couple of times already, asking for an update on Michael's condition.

When Dr. Sampler got the report of the spinal fluid chemistry, he saw that the protein was elevated, the sugar was decreased, and the lymphocytes (white blood cells) were increased.

"Laura, I have to put Michael on Amphotericin. All the findings on the spinal fluid suggest fungus infection."

"Do whatever you think is best, Dr. Sampler."

Dr. Sampler took Laura aside.

"I don't think you will even have time to take Michael home. He is too sick. He can succumb into a coma anytime. Let's wait for forty-eight hours to see how he responds to the antibiotics."

"Do whatever you think is best for Michael."

It was almost five o'clock and Laura had not heard from Jeanie or Mrs. Secula. Dr. Simmons was still there.

"Dr. Simmons, I think you better go home. You must be very tired."

"Laura, I have nothing to do at home but read. I might as well stay with you and Michael."

The nurse came in to take Michael's vital signs. His temperature was 102°, his pulse was 110/min, and his blood pressure was stable.

Laura looked at Dr. Simmons. There was sadness evident in Dr. Simmons' face. He, too, was trying to control his emotions. Laura took Michael's hand and grasped it.

"Michael, how are you feeling?"

"Laura, it feels like my whole body is on fire. My head is pounding. I wish God would take me now. I feel very frustrated and very tired. I know I am about to lose everything I love. Laura, please hold my hand. I want to hold Jennifer, too. Is Father John coming?"

"He will be coming soon."

The head nurse from the ICU came to see Laura. "Dr. Secula, there is a phone call for you at the nurses' station."

"Michael, Dr. Simmons, I will just see who is on the phone."

"I will stay with Michael."

It was Mrs. Secula on the phone.

"Laura, we are at the airport. We are waiting for the arrival of Father John. We will go to the hospital from the airport."

"Mom, please hurry. I think Michael might lapse into coma soon. I am so helpless and frustrated. I am a physician and I cannot even help Michael!"

"Laura, I understand your frustration. But we have to trust God. Everything happens for a reason."

"I know, Mom, but sometimes the truth is very hard to accept. I hope Michael will still be able to communicate when you arrive."

"I hope so, too."

"Mom, I have to go back to Michael's room. I will see you later. How is Jennifer?"

"Jennifer is fine."

"Michael wants to hold Jennifer. I hope Dr. Sampler lets him hold Jennifer for one last time."

"I hope so, too."

"Goodbye, Mom."

Laura went back to Michael's room. Dr. Simmons was dozing when she arrived.

"Dr. Simmons, do you want to have dinner?"

"No, Laura. I have no appetite. How about you? Do you want to go to dinner in the cafeteria?"

"No, Dr. Simmons. I would rather stay with Michael. I just talked to my mother. Jeanie, Mom, and Jennifer are all in the airport waiting for Father John's arrival."

"I don't know how Father John will react when he sees Michael in this condition."

"I am sure he will be shocked and saddened at the same time."

"I can understand that; he raised Michael himself."

Thirty minutes later, Laura and Dr. Simmons were surprised to see Father John and Mrs. Secula at Michael's doorway. Jeanie and Jennifer were waiting at the information desk.

"Michael, it's Father John. How are you feeling?"

"I feel weak and frustrated, Father John. I cannot even see you. I lost my vision this morning. Everything is going too fast for me. I am very tired. I just want to go to sleep now."

"Michael, please don't say that. We are all here to give you moral support," sobbed Laura.

"Laura, I hope you don't forget about our discussion of dying. I will always watch over you and Jennifer. I wish I could hold Jennifer before I go."

"Dr. Sampler is not here to give his permission."

Father John gave Michael his last rites.

Laura was at the left side of the bed and was holding Michael's hand tightly. All of a sudden, Michael's grasp became loose.

"Michael, oh, Michael! Michael! Oh, my God!, we just lost him!"

The nurses rushed to Michael's room.

Laura quietly said to them, "No code please."

The nurses went back to the nurses' station. The head nurse notified the supervisor. Laura remained stoic throughout. She remained in Michael's room until the morgue stretcher arrived for Michael's body. Special precautions had to be used. Laura looked tired, downhearted, and shocked. Michael's death had not sunk into her yet. Her face was practically expressionless. She could not even cry. She remained very quiet. Father John and Mrs. Secula came back to the room to get Laura. Dr. Simmons stayed with Jennifer and Jeanie downstairs in the lobby.

"Laura, you look very pale and hungry. Do you want anything to eat?"

"No, Father John. I would rather go home. Where is Dr. Simmons?"

"He is with Jennifer and Jeanie."

"I want to see him and talk to him. He was here the whole day with me. He has been so good to me and Michael. I don't know how I will ever be able to repay his kindness."

As soon as Laura saw Dr. Simmons, she started crying.

"Dr. Simmons, you have been so good to me and Michael. I don't know what we would have done without all your help and support."

"Laura, I try to help all my friends. I always considered Michael one of my sons. He was a very nice and a caring person. I am going to miss him. I am going home now. I will have to call James Dillon, John Miller, and Estela and Jorge. I will call you tomorrow about your funeral plans. If you need anything, don't hesitate to call me."

"Thank you, Dr. Simmons."

Dr. Simmons kissed Mrs. Secula, Laura, Jeanie, and Jennifer. He shook Father John's hand.

"Father John, you raised a very wonderful man. We will all miss him. He is a big loss to the medical profession."

"We will be seeing you, Dr. Simmons."

Laura and her family left soon after Dr. Simmons. Laura took Jennifer from Jeanie. She was trying to hold back her tears.

"Laura, I will drive. Just leave your car in the parking lot."

"Jeanie, I will be able to drive. Father John will ride with me in my car. Jennifer and Mom will ride with you."

"Laura, I will drive. You are too upset to be able to concentrate on your driving."

"Thank you, Father John."

The drive home seemed an eternity for Laura. Once they got in the car, Laura started crying.

"I am sorry, Father John. I just cannot control myself anymore. I just have to cry."

"I understand, Laura. I am in shock, too. Michael died too fast. I guess, though, that's for the best."

As soon an they arrived at Kalina St., Laura went up to the kitchen to see if there was any food left for Father John.

"Father John, it is almost four o'clock in the morning. Do you want breakfast?"

"No, I will just drink a glass of milk."

Jeanie pulled into the driveway. Jennifer was already asleep in the arms of Mrs. Secula.

"I have to put Jennifer to bed. She is very tired. Father John, please make yourself comfortable. You can sleep in the third bedroom. Everything is ready for you. Please get some rest."

"I will as soon as I finish drinking my milk. Laura, do you want to talk?"

"Father, please, get some sleep. I will talk to you later. I have to rest myself, too."

Jeanie went to bed. Laura and Mrs. Secula were left in the kitchen.

"Mom, how did you deal with Dad's death?"

"I prayed. I knew that life must go on. It helped me very much that I had you and Jeanie, the best daughters that a Mom could ever ask for. You were both very supportive of me. Your concern for me was overwhelming. I could not help but get myself out of the depression."

"Thanks, Mom. Michael always told me that death is a positive sign of living. Michael has taught us all how to die with dignity."

"Laura, let's get some sleep. You have to think of the funeral arrangements you will make tomorrow."

"I also have to call all the AIDS patients Michael called regularly. I want them to know that Michael is gone and that he was thinking of them until the end. I want to let them know that Michael really cared about them."

CHAPTER XXXIII

It was already eleven o'clock when Laura got up. She had tossed in bed the whole night. She hardly slept. She cried the whole night. Her eyes were red and swollen. She felt very weak.

"Laura, please try to eat. You are going to get sick."

"Mom, I have no appetite. I feel like I have died, too. I feel like a part of me has been cut off and taken away."

"Laura, I understand what you feel, but you have to look at it this way. Everything happens for a purpose. God knows why he took away Michael so soon. We have to accept God's will."

"Mom, I understand. But I am in so much pain right now that I cannot think straight. My emotions are overwhelming my mind. I have to pray very hard for acceptance. Where is Father John?"

"He is still asleep. He must be very tired, too."

"Mom, I am going downstairs. I am going to call the funeral home."

Laura called the funeral director. Laura decided on a closed casket with no viewing. There would be a mass before the funeral, and the burial would be at Ascension Cemetery. There would be no announcement in the obituary section of the newspaper. The funeral would be on November 18, 1985. Laura called Dr. Simmons and Debbie to tell them about the funeral arrangement.

"I just finished talking to Jorge, Estela, and John Miller. They will be coming for the funeral. Laura, please don't hesitate to call me if you need anything."

"Thank you, Dr. Simmons."

Laura called Michael's friends in an AIDS rooming house. She told them that Michael was gone and that he died in peace.

"I am sorry to hear that. We lost a good friend in Michael."

"I know, and I lost my best friend and husband. You can call me if you need help. Michael's friends are also my friends."

"Thank you, Mrs. Olsire."

"You are welcome."

Laura went back upstairs to see if Father John and Jennifer were awake. Jennifer was still sleeping. Father John was having breakfast.

"Laura, how are you holding up?"

"I am fine, Father John. We have to go to St. Archangel's Church to talk to the parish priest. We have to ask his permission for you to say the Requiem Mass for Michael."

"Laura, why don't you eat breakfast now?"

"I am not hungry, Father. I will have coffee. Father Walls said that we could talk to him after mass this afternoon. Please, get some rest after you finish breakfast. I will call our relatives in South Philadelphia while I am waiting for Jennifer to wake up."

By the time Laura finished calling her relatives in South Philadelphia, Jennifer was awake. Laura took Jennifer with her to feed her. After Jennifer finished eating, Laura bathed her.

Jennifer was a little bit cranky. She must have been tired. She could probably sense her Mom's sadness, too, but could not express it yet! It was almost time for Jennifer's nap after her bath. Laura tucked her in bed again. After Jennifer had fallen asleep, Laura went down to the basement to sort out and pack Michael's clothes.

Laura tried to lie down and rest, but she was just overcome with grief. She just lay still and cried and cried until it was time for her to go to church with Father John. She felt very weak. Her knees were wobbly. She tried to eat, but she still did not have an appetite.

"Laura, are you sure you want to go to church with us? Your mom and I can talk to Father Walls. You don't have to come if you feel weak."

"I will be fine, Father."

The five of them went to Saturday mass. Jeanie drove. After church, they went to the sacristy to talk to Father Walls. Father Walls was very understanding and went along with all their plans.

As soon as the Seculas and Father John arrived home, they had dinner.

"Laura, please try to eat something. You might get sick."

"I will try my best."

Laura hardly ate, but she did drink orange juice and eat her soup. She asked to be excused and took Jennifer with her down to the basement. She played with Jennifer and showed her pictures of Michael. Jennifer smiled whenever she saw Michael's picture.

"Jennifer, this is Daddy, but he is now gone. He is watching over us in heaven."

Laura and Jennifer both fell asleep. Mrs. Secula and Jeanie came down to see how Laura and Jennifer were doing. They did not want to disturb them. Jeanie and Mrs. Secula went upstairs to see how Father John was doing. He was already in his room.

On Sunday morning, the Seculas and Father John just stayed home. Laura was in bed practically the whole day.

Mrs. Secula went down to the basement to talk to Laura.

"Laura, you have to get hold of yourself. You cannot go on living like this. You must realize you have Jennifer to raise. The poor little girl does not even know that her Daddy died."

"Mom, I think we are underestimating Jennifer. I think she can sense that Michael is gone."

"Laura, come up and eat with us. You might not have enough strength to withstand the funeral tomorrow."

"Thanks, Mom. I will be up."

Laura tried to eat as much as she could. After dinner, everyone went to bed early so that they would all get enough rest for tomorrow's mass and funeral.

Everyone was up early. Most of the relatives of the Seculas from South Philadelphia had arrived. They would have to go to the funeral parlor first. By nine o'clock, the funeral cortege was already at St. Archangel's Church. The Seculas and Father John were seated in the front row. At ten o'clock, Father John said the mass and the eulogy. He made mention of the fact that he baptized Michael, raised him, married him, and now was going to bury him. Everyone listened as he extolled Michael as a man and as a physician. Everyone was misty-eyed. Laura tried to control her emotions as she listened attentively to what Father John was saying.

The trip to Ascension Cemetery was short. Everyone placed a red rose on top of Michael's casket. Father John said some prayers, too, before the casket was lowered. Father John invited everyone for lunch at the Secula residence before everyone left the cemetery.

The Simmonses, Cortezes, Millers, and most of the Seculas' relatives went to the house for lunch.

Practically everyone was gone by five o'clock. All the doctors stayed behind to express their condolences to the family.

"Laura, if you need us for anything, please do not hesitate to call us."

"I will. Thank you for all your kindness to me and Michael. Dr. Simmons, you really had made our load lighter. Just knowing that you and Debbie would be available whenever Michael and I needed your help made a world of difference. I cannot thank you enough."

Laura hugged everyone on their way out. "Thanks again."

"Remember, Laura, keep in touch."

"I will."

It was noticeable to them that none of Laura's co-residents came to the funeral. Laura had wanted it that way. She did not want Dr. Scoop to find out anything about Michael's illness and death.

Father John stayed for a couple of days before he left for Indiana. All the Seculas took him to the airport. He hugged each one.

"Laura, please pray. Call me anytime you feel like talking."

"I will, Father John, and thank you for everything."

Father John hurriedly boarded the plane. He could see that Laura was getting misty-eyed. Jennifer had fallen asleep in Mrs. Secula's arms.

In a couple of days, it would be Thanksgiving. The Seculas had completely forgotten about the coming festivity.

"Mom, why don't we drop by the supermarket and get our turkey?"

"Well, Jeanie, go on in, if you want, and we will wait for you in the car. I really don't feel like cooking anything after this tragedy, though."

"You are right, Mom."

"Listen, you two. I understand, but, knowing Michael, I think he would want us to have turkey dinner. He is watching over us."

"You're right, Laura. I will go into the supermarket then."

"It's on the next block."

Finally, Jeanie parked at Creden St. near the supermarket. Jeanie went inside the store. There was a long line of people in each of the register areas. Each one of them had bought a turkey and trimmings. Jeanie took the last turkey. It was almost lunch time by the time the Seculas arrived home.

"Laura, you must eat. Jennifer needs you."

"I will just lie down for a while, Mom. I feel very tired. I guess I am depressed. I know I have to help myself. I have not really cried enough."

"Why don't you eat something before you sleep?"

"I guess I have to. Let me feed Jennifer, too."

The three of them hardly ate. Laura went downstairs to rest. Jennifer was tucked in bed by Jeanie.

It was almost five o'clock when Mrs. Secula went down to see how Laura was doing. Laura was fitfully sleeping. Her face was a picture of sadness. Her brows were arched and she looked pale and haggard. She had not put on make-up since Michael's death. Mrs. Secula just sat near the study table and watched Laura as she tossed in bed. She picked up some of the clothes that Laura was trying to sort out.

By six-thirty, Laura finally woke up.

"Mom, I am sorry I overslept. I was so exhausted. My headache is practically gone now."

"I am glad, Laura. Do you want to bake pumpkin pie for tomorrow?"

"Whatever you want to do, Mom."

Laura called her senior resident.

"How are you, Laura?"

"I am fine. Is Dr. Scoop still around?"

"He just left, but he will be here tomorrow in spite of the holiday."

"How come?"

"We have a couple of sick patients. I expect him to be here by ten o'clock."

"I will give him a call then. Thank you."

Laura and Mrs. Secula went upstairs to have dinner. Jeanie had already fed Jennifer. She was almost ready to be put to bed. Laura took Jennifer from Jeanie. Laura hugged Jennifer.

"I'm glad you can't understand what is going on."

Jennifer just looked at her Mom. Jeanie took Jennifer and put her to bed.

Laura and Mrs. Secula talked for a while.

"Michael and I were so happy until AIDS attacked his body and mind. My heart is aching, overwhelmed by emptiness, grief and sorrow; a part of me has been taken away abruptly. I know God will grant me the strength and courage to accept His will. He will give me strength to carry on and to raise Jennifer the way Michael would have wanted her raised."

"Laura, you will be fine. You have a strong faith which will help you pull through this grief and loss. It will take time, but you will be able to do it. Trust me."

Laura stood up and hugged her Mom. "Mom, I have to go to bed now. I have to call Dr. Scoop tomorrow."

Laura woke up very early. She went upstairs and cooked breakfast. She got dressed and went to St. Archangel's Church to hear mass. It was almost nine o'clock when she got back. Jeanie, Mrs. Secula, and Jennifer were just finishing breakfast. Laura ate her cereal and drank a cup of coffee.

"Mom, I want to go to the cemetery to visit Michael."

"We can all go then."

"I just have to call Dr. Scoop at ten o'clock. After I call him, we can all go."

"I will just bathe and change Jennifer's dress."

At exactly ten o'clock, Laura called the surgical department. Dr. Scoop was already in the hospital.

Dr. Scoop got on the phone.

"Laura, I heard you called me yesterday. What for?"

"Dr. Scoop, I am ready to come back to work."

"So soon? How is your husband?"

"He died suddenly. His brain was affected."

"Well, as I have said to you on the phone, you will have to get HIV and Western Blot tests. You can have it done tomorrow. It takes ten days to two weeks to get the results. If they are negative, you can come back after the first week of December. I am sorry to hear about the death of your husband."

"Thank you, Dr. Scoop."

Laura hung up the phone and said, "Let's go, Mom. Is Jennifer already dressed?"

"Jennifer and I will be down shortly."

It did not take them that long to reach Ascension Cemetery. The cemetery was practically empty. There were only a few people visiting their loved ones. As soon as they reached the site where Michael was buried, Laura got very upset.

"All the fresh bouquets of roses that we left are all gone. It's only been a few days since Michael was buried. I cannot understand this! Do scavengers pick up flowers in the cemetery and sell them in the streets?"

"Laura, don't get too upset about things you have no control over."

"But, Mom, those roses were in flower pots, and the rose bushes had roots!"

"There is nothing we can do about it. We will just have to bring flowers next time."

"People have no respect for the dead."

"When will Michael's tombstone be put in?"

"In two weeks."

After the Seculas had prayed, they quietly left. It was lunch time when they arrived home. Mrs. Secula put the turkey in the oven. Jeanie fed Jennifer. Laura went down to the basement to finish sorting out Michael's clothes. She would have to dispose of all of Michael's clothes through the infectious waste company. She went upstairs and had a light lunch with Jeanie and her Mom.

Before they sat down for their Thanksgiving dinner, Laura tried to call Father John, but he was not in the convent.

Dinner was quiet, to the point of being solemn. Everyone was thinking of Michael. Jennifer was trying to grab some of the cookies from her high chair. She had her eyes fixed on the chair where Michael used to sit during dinner time. Laura kept her eyes on Jennifer.

After dinner, Laura helped Jeanie with the dishes. Mrs. Secula bathed and tucked Jennifer into bed.

Laura woke up early. She cooked breakfast for everyone. She was going to Northend Hospital to get her blood testing for AIDS. She went directly to the pathologist's office.

"I am sorry to hear about your husband's death. That was a shame. He was at the prime of his life."

"Thank you, Dr. Seawell, but I would prefer not to talk about it. I am not ready to discuss it with anyone. Besides, there is litigation going on about this AIDS case."

"I am sorry, Laura."

"Thank you, Dr. Seawell."

"I will give you a call as soon as I get the test results. Where can I reach you?"

"I will be home. I was instructed by Dr. Scoop not to come to work until I get my test results."

"I will call you at home then."

"I will be expecting your call soon. Thank you, Dr. Seawell."

Laura did not go to the ward to see her co-residents. She went directly home. She had a lot of things to do in the basement. She had to write thank-you notes to all the people who had come to the mass and funeral.

Days had passed and she still had not heard from Dr. Seawell. On the fourteenth day after her tests, she called his office.

"Dr. Seawell is no longer working here."

"How come?"

"I don't know."

"Well, I would like to know if you have received the report of my test."

"It should be in tomorrow."

"I will call you back tomorrow. Whom shall I ask for?"

"Just ask for me."

"What is your name?"

"Sarah James."

"Thank you, Sarah. I will call you tomorrow then."

"Have a nice day."

"You, too."

Laura could not sleep that night. She was worried about her test result. She lay awake all night. "Dear God, please help me. Jennifer needs someone to take care of her."

The next morning, Laura woke up early. She waited until nine o'clock to call Sarah James. She was put on hold because Sarah James was on the other line.

"Hello, is this Dr. Secula? I have good news for you. Your tests are both negative. I am happy for you."

"Please send a copy of that report to Dr. Scoop. I will call him as soon as I hang up. Thank you so much and thank you for caring."

As soon as Laura hung up, she went upstairs and told Mrs. Secula. Jennifer was just having her breakfast. She looked playful and cheerful today.

"Jennifer, how is your breakfast?"

Jennifer just smiled at her Mom, showing her two small teeth.

Laura would be going back to work in a couple of days. She called Smithsvale Hospital to see if there was an opening in the accident ward. She took the dates of the open slot to see if it was in conflict with her night duty at Northend Hospital.

Laura called Dr. Scoop in the afternoon to see if she could get the night call schedule. Dr. Scoop told her to get in touch with Dr. Saltine. He gave her the list of the dates she was on and off. Laura would be working Christmas Eve. There was nothing Laura could do about the schedule during the Christmas holidays. She had to compensate for the days she had taken off while Michael was sick. It dawned on Laura that Christmas was almost approaching. No matter how grief-stricken she was, she decided to go shopping with Mrs. Secula to buy Jennifer a Christmas outfit and some toys. She brought some presents for her Mom and Jeanie, too. Laura decided to work two nights a week at the emergency room at Smithsvale Hospital. Southern Hospital was not doing well at all because of the Medicare suspension imposed on them in the past. The hospital was about to declare bankruptcy under Chapter 11.

Christmas came and went. The Seculas did not celebrate it as they usually did. Mrs. Secula did not put out all her Christmas decorations. They decided to put up a tree for Jennifer. Laura called Father John to wish him a happy holiday.

Laura worked regularly in the two hospitals. Her renovation loan had been paid off. She was trying to save some money to go on vacation with her Mom and Jeanie. Mrs. Secula advised her to go with Debbie instead to Miami in April to visit Jorge and Estela.

"Laura, I think you should go with Debbie to Miami in April. You need to relax. Jeanie and I will take care of Jennifer."

"But I don't want to impose on you and Jeanie. You have done enough for me already."

"Laura, you need to get away and relax. You have been working too much. Debbie and Estela have invited you to come down to Miami, and I think you should go. Anyway, it would be after Jennifer's birthday. Sometimes, you have to think of yourself, too. You have been brooding practically everyday. I am sure Michael would want you to go on living. I know you are in a lot of emotional pain, but you have to be realistic, too. You have to go on with your life. Jennifer needs you. You have to relax and take care of yourself. You might get sick. You have not done anything for yourself since Michael died. All you do is work, work, work! That's why I think you should go to Miami with Debbie in April."

"I will think about it, Mom."

CHAPTER XXXIV

Jennifer had her first birthday party on April 13, 1986. She did not have any cousins her age. Her guests were mostly adults from South Philadelphia, Debbie, and Dr. Simmons. Clapping her hands, Jennifer blew out her one candle and at the same time delightedly said her first syllables, "Da da." Tears welled up in Laura's eyes. She took Jennifer and hugged her. Jennifer reciprocated with a twinkle in her eyes. Mrs. Secula watched the interaction between Jennifer and Laura. She, too, could not control her emotions. Laura finally cut Jennifer's cake and gave each of the twenty-five guests a piece.

"Michael would have been so proud of Jennifer if he were here," whispered Jeanie to Mrs. Secula. Mrs. Secula nodded.

Everyone sang "Happy Birthday" to Jennifer. Jennifer was thrilled to see everyone giving her their undivided attention. She clapped her hands, too, and squealed at the top of her little voice.

Everyone loved the pound cake Mrs. Secula had baked. It had taken her two days to bake such a big cake.

It was almost six o'clock when most of the guests left. Debbie and Dr. Simmons stayed to talk to Laura to finalize their trip to Miami, Florida.

"Laura, how many weeks vacation were you able to take?"

"Just one week. I just need time to sort out my life. I don't want to be away from Jennifer for too long. I will sorely miss her."

"Laura, don't worry about Jennifer. Mom and I will take good care of her."

"Thanks, Jeanie. I know both you and Mom love Jennifer very much."

"Laura, we will pick you up on the 15th of April at eight o'clock in the morning. Jorge and Estela will be waiting for us at the airport. They are quite disappointed that Jennifer is not coming with us. Nedda is anxious to meet her."

"Well, someday Nedda and Jennifer will meet each other."

"We will see you then. Mrs. Secula, thank you for inviting us."

"Thank you for coming and for all your kindness to Laura and Jennifer."

Debbie and Dr. Simmons finally left.

Laura went to her room and Jennifer's to start her packing. She went through all her clothes. She was going to take only a few wash-and-wear clothes to save space in her luggage. After she finished packing, she went back to the kitchen to help clean the dishes and straighten up.

"Laura, please try to enjoy yourself down in Miami. I know you need this rest very badly. You look very tired and worn out."

Ring===Ring===Ring

Laura picked up the phone. It was Father John. He was calling to wish Jennifer a "Happy Birthday" and to see how Laura was doing.

"Father John, thank you for thinking of us. Jennifer just had her first birthday celebration today. The guests just left a little while ago. She said her first syllables today as well. I wish you were here. You would have been proud of your granddaughter."

"I wish I could talk to her. Someday, she will find out that her father was a kind and gentle person."

"She will definitely learn more about Michael, Father, once she is old enough to understand. I intend to instill in her Michael's sense of values. She will really have a good role model. Father, do you want to talk to my mother?"

"Yes, please."

Laura handed the phone to her mom.

"Mrs. Secula, how are you?"

"We are all fine, Father. I wish you would come and visit us."

"I would love to do that once my assistant pastor gets better. Right now, his diabetes is still out of control."

"Well, let us know, Father, when you are available. We would love to have you here. I am sure Jennifer would be happy to see you, too."

"That would be nice. May I speak to Laura again, please."

Mrs. Secula put Laura on the phone.

"Laura, how are you holding up?"

"I am doing fine, Father. Sometimes, I feel a lot of pain and anguish, but I don't think I am in a deep depression. I pray a lot. I try to live one day at a time. It is hard emotionally, but my faith keeps me going. Life must go on. Jennifer needs me!"

"That is what I wanted to hear from you, Laura."

"Just pray for me, Father John."

"I do all the time. I am sure Michael is watching over you, too."

"I know. There are days that I ask him to pray for me, too."

"Well, Laura, take care of yourself and Jennifer. You both are always in my prayers."

"Thank you, Father. We look forward to seeing you in the future. Goodbye."

"Goodbye, Laura."

On April 15, 1986, Debbie and Dr. Simmons picked up Laura on their way to the airport. Jennifer started crying when she saw her mother leaving. Laura ran back upstairs and gave Jennifer a kiss and a tight hug. She could not help but cry as well. She wished she could take Jennifer with her.

The trip to the airport was a leisurely drive. The Schuylkill Expressway was empty. Very few cars were on the street. Being a Saturday morning, half of the people in Philadelphia were probably still sleeping.

As soon as they arrived at the airport, they heard the loudspeaker announcing the flight numbers of different planes going to different parts of the country. Flight 056 was leaving at 9:15 a.m.. Debbie and Laura went to the boarding gate and bade Dr. Simmons goodbye. Dr. Simmons left for home as soon as the plane took off.

As soon as Laura and Debbie got settled in their seats, the stewardess started giving safety flight instructions. Afterwards, the stewardesses distributed some snacks and sodas.

The flight to Miami was quite smooth. Although they had two stopovers, they arrived in Miami on time. They saw Jorge and Estela waving at them as soon as they alighted from the plane. Jorge and Estela were delighted to see them.

Once they all got into the car, Jorge broke the silence.

"I have to tell you something very important which Estela could not tell you on the phone or write about."

"What is it, Jorge?"

"Before Michael died, I had a long discussion with him about Ditas getting a job here in Florida in a health spa and weight-reducing facility owned by a Florida lawyer and a doctor. Well, this health spa is not what it should be."

"In what sense?" asked Debbie.

"It houses a drug-ring. Ditas and the other five girls recruited from the Pineapple Republic were being used as conduits for money laundering."

"In what way?" a stunned Laura asked.

"Well, twice a week they deposited hundred and hundreds of thousands of dollars into the National Pineapple Bank via telegraphic deposit to the Milagrosa Bank. This money in turn was deposited by the National Pineapple Bank into a Switzerland bank. From Switzerland, it was transferred back to the Milagrosa Bank here in Miami."

"So, where is Ditas now?"

"Ditas is under the protective custody of the FBI here in Miami."

"How did that come about?"

Before Jorge could answer, he realized that he had passed by their house. He had to drive around the block of Martinique Street to get to his driveway. He took the luggage of Debbie and Laura.

"Estela, I will just park the car in the garage. As soon as Laura and Debbie are done unpacking, we can go out to eat."

"Jorge, we prefer to stay in so that we can continue our conversation about Ditas' plight," said Laura and Debbie in unison.

"Whatever you want. You are our guests. We will just stay in the house for dinner then. We can eat take-out."

Debbie and Laura unpacked their luggage and took showers. It was almost dinner time by the time they were finished.

Estela had already called their favorite restaurant to deliver some food to their house. She heated some chicken wings and fish sticks for Debbie and Laura to nibble on while they were awaiting the food from the restaurant. Estela had also set the table exquisitely with a flower arrangement from her own garden and greenhouse. Finally, the food from the restaurant was delivered. Estela called everyone to take their places at the dining table. Nedda had been fed early by her nanny. She was now playing in her playroom with her nanny.

Everyone said grace.

"Jorge, let's go back to our conversation about Ditas. How did she get into the custody of the FBI?"

"Well, last month we got a letter from Ditas which was mailed for her by a teller of Milagrosa Bank. The teller did not have any idea of the content of the envelope."

"What was the letter all about?"

Jorge stood up and said, "I will get it from the library. I kept it for both of you to take home. It might help your medico-legal malpractice case. I have another authenticated copy which Ditas might need once the FBI zeroes in on Robert Smith."

"Robert Smith!!! Is he the same Robert Smith from Philadelphia?"

"I am not sure, but Ditas sent a calling card with the letter and it does have a Philadelphia address."

Jorge went to the library to get Ditas' letter. He handed the envelope to Debbie.

"Laura, do you remember the address of the Robert Smith who filed the lawsuit against Dad, Michael, and the others?"

"No, but we can find out when we get home. Even if there are about twenty lawyers with this name, we can still single him out if we have his address."

"That would be marvelous. This will help us start our own sting operation against him."

"I hope so."

Jorge continued, "Once we got Ditas' letter, I contacted the chief of the FBI in Miami who, by coincidence, happens to be my patient. That made things easier for us. One day, early in the morning, the FBI agents nabbed Ditas, while she was depositing money, and took custody of her. The FBI agents were unable to nab Ditas' companion because there was a shootout in the bank between the FBI agents and the Sampaguita drug cartel. Ditas' friend is now either being held as a hostage in Robert Smith's mansion or, more likely, is probably buried in his backyard."

"Why do you say that?"

"After Ditas was nabbed, the Sampaguita cartel, Robert Smith, and his doctor friend remained on the Mabini yacht docked in Key West, Florida. The FBI agents obtained a search warrant and went to the mansion. They found body parts in the freezer: a human brain, pancreas, spleen, liver, and kidneys. They dug in the backyard where there were newly put in sods. The fresh sods were actually covering the graves of four young women. Ditas confirmed the presence of these human bodies. One time at midnight, when she was staying at the mansion, she had awakened and, by chance, had looked out in the backyard. She saw Robert Smith and the doctor digging the graves. The bodies were just wrapped in plastic sheets. This incident made Ditas realize that she and the other girl would be the next victims. She made a fast move by befriending the teller at the bank. She is very sorry that the other girl didn't make it out with her."

"How were the FBI agents able to search the mansion?"

"They obtained a search warrant first. Then, the FBI agents sent some reconnaissance planes to watch the yacht while they were searching the mansion and installing monitoring devices."

"How clever."

"I was surprised that Ditas was still able to think straight with the tension and pressure she was going through."

"What will happen to Ditas now?"

"She will be under the protective custody of the FBI. After the trial, she will not be able to go back to the Pineapple Republic. Ditas will have to go under the Federal Witness Protection program."

"I hope the Sampaguita Cartel doesn't find out where she is now."

"Is there a chance we can talk to her?"

"No, she is incommunicado right now."

"How about taking us around town? You can probably show us the mansion of Robert Smith."

"I would be afraid to do that. The Sampaguita Cartel might have some surveillance monitors on the roof. We would be jeopardizing our lives."

"You're right. It was a stupid idea. I am sorry for even suggesting it, Jorge."

"That's alright, Debbie. I understand what you are trying to do. You are trying to help the case of your dad against Robert Smith."

"Thank you for understanding, Jorge."

"You are welcome, Debbie."

It was almost eleven o'clock in the evening when everyone went to bed. Debbie was restless. Robert Smith's face kept on flashing into her mind. She made up her mind to see the District Attorney of Philadelphia as soon as she got home.

On Sunday, they attended the ten o'clock mass and went to a restaurant for brunch. After brunch, Jorge and Estela showed Debbie and Laura around. On Sunday night, Jorge, Estela,

Laura, and Debbie went out to dinner. They were busy talking when a tall, stern-looking man passed by with a young Spanish-looking girl. Jorge whispered to Estela.

"That's Robert Smith with Ditas' co-worker! I wonder what he is up to now?"

"You are right, Jorge. I have seen him before! I hope he does not hurt that girl!" Laura exclaimed.

"I hope so, too."

At eleven o'clock, Robert Smith and his companion left. Jorge and everyone watched where Robert Smith was heading. He headed towards the beach. The companion of Robert Smith looked dazed when they left.

Jorge, Laura, Estela, and Debbie arrived home by midnight. They did not talk long. Everyone was tired.

"Jorge, you don't have to take off from your schedule. Laura and I would prefer to stay home and talk to Estela. We also want to get acquainted with Nedda. Gee, I forgot to give you Nedda's present!"

"Whatever you want to do is fine with us."

"Good night, everyone."

Laura and Debbie talked about Robert Smith before they went to bed.

"Laura, is the Robert Smith we saw at the restaurant the same Robert Smith who deposed everyone that day?"

"Yes, we have to do our own investigation fast. We have to stop this shark. What do you plan to do, Debbie?"

"I have to meet with the District Attorney in Philadelphia to see if he will help us nail him."

"That's a good idea."

"We better sleep now so we can develop our strategy. Good night, Laura."

"Good night, Debbie."

Estela, Debbie, and Laura were having breakfast when their attention was caught by a flash report on the television. "The body of a young Spanish girl was found in Miami Beach at twelve-thirty Monday morning."

Laura, Debbie, and Estela were stunned when the picture of the girl was shown.

"She was Ditas' companion! That's the one we saw last night! I have to call Jorge so that he can notify the FBI chief."

"Robert Smith must have killed that girl, too, because she knew too much."

"He probably did."

"God, the situation is getting worse! We better be careful. He might get us killed, too, if he knew we were on to him."

"Laura, do you think he saw and recognized you in the restaurant?"

"I don't think so. I don't think he would have remembered me."

"Well, we still have to be careful."

"I know. This guy is unpredictable and irrational."

Ring===Ring===Ring

When Estela answered the phone, she heard a familiar voice.

"Hello, this is Dr. Simmons."

"Dr. Simmons, this is Estela! How are you? We were hoping that you would come down with Debbie and Laura."

"I have no time right now. I am researching our medical malpractice suit. I am calling to tell Debbie and Laura that we are going to trial April 27, 1986. This is quite sudden. It has only been a little more than two years since this case was first filed. I can't understand why we are going on trial so soon. I think Robert Smith is in with the legal justice system in Philadelphia, too. He must have some judges on his payroll."

"I would not be surprised if he did. Well, here is Debbie."

When Estela handed Debbie the phone, Dr. Simmons said, "Debbie, I think you and Laura should come home now. I need help to research AIDS. I have already called James Dillon and John Miller. They will both be flying in two days before the trial. Two days should be enough time for James to get over his jet lag."

"Laura and I will fly back a soon as we can. I will call the airlines as soon as I hang up. Laura and I talked about this case last night. We both agree that we should do our own investigation to stop this man. I want to get his business partner's name. He is a doctor. I think Smith uses this doctor as his hired gun on all his medical malpractice cases."

"I would not be surprised. Call me as soon as your flight is finalized."

Debbie called the airlines. She was able to get a flight for Tuesday at two o'clock in the afternoon.

She called back Dr. Simmons.

"Dad, Laura and I will be flying home tomorrow at two o'clock in the afternoon. We will be waiting for you at the airport. Please call Laura's mom, but don't tell her the real reason for cutting our vacation short. Just tell her I have some important autopsies to do in the coroner's office. Please tell her we will drive Laura home after dinner. We have so many things to talk about. Take care, Dad."

"Take care, Debbie."

The next morning, Debbie, Laura, and Estela woke up early. The morning paper carried this headline: "The FBI office took over the investigation of the drowning of a young Spanish girl who used to work for attorney, Robert Smith. Robert Smith was questioned, but he denied any knowledge or involvement in the death of the girl. He was very upset with the questioning of the FBI agents."

After breakfast, Laura and Debbie started packing their bags. Debbie confirmed their flights. Laura and Debbie played with Nedda for a while. They both talked to Jorge before lunch and thanked him for their hospitality.

"Thank you for Ditas' letter. I think we can use it against Robert Smith. I also cut out the news account of the death of that young Spanish girl. I hope it will help our case."

"I hope so, too, Debbie. I will keep you posted on her drowning."

"Thanks, Jorge."

Laura added, "Jorge, thanks, too, for all you've done for us."

Estela drove Laura and Debbie to the airport. Estela was sad to see them leave so soon.

CHAPTER XXXV

Dr. Simmons was already at Philadelphia airport when Laura and Debbie got off the plane. He waited for them at the baggage claim department.

The three of them ate dinner at the Bellevue before they took Laura home. They discussed Robert Smith and the drowning case in Miami. Debbie intended to go to the FBI office with Laura as soon as Laura located the two letters Charlie had left for Michael. They hoped the letters would incriminate Robert Smith somehow. They had only ten days left before the medical malpractice trial started.

By nine o'clock, they were at the Secula residence. Mrs. Secula and Jennifer were still awake. Jennifer squealed when she saw Laura. Laura took Jennifer from Mrs. Secula. Dr. Simmons and Debbie both kissed Jennifer.

As soon as Debbie and Dr. Simmons left, Laura went down to the basement. She looked all over for Charlie's letters. She could not find the box where the florigraphy books were kept. She went over all the stacked-up boxes. The florigraphy box was at the bottom of the stack. She reached for all the florigraphy books. Finally, she found the two letters. She did not know whether she should open them now or not. She decided to call Debbie.

"Debbie, do you think I should open these letters now?"

"Laura, please don't open them now; otherwise, the FBI chief might consider them invalid. We will use these letters to convince the chief of the FBI office in Philadelphia to meet with us. I will tell him when I call him tomorrow that, since the letters are a death-bed confession, they might contain some information about Robert Smith who got Charlie hooked on drugs. I will let you know when we will see him. In the meantime, do you think you can help Dad do research on the most current information about AIDS?"

"I will be glad to."

"Good night, Laura."

"Good night, Debbie."

Laura went upstairs. Mrs. Secula had already tucked Jennifer in bed.

"Laura, why are you so jittery?"

"The lawsuit of Patty Singleton is going on trial April 27, 1986."

"Why so soon?"

"I don't know, Mom. Robert Smith must have all the right legal connections."

"Well, I don't think he will prevail on this case. He hasn't a leg to stand on."

"I hope so, Mom. I might be called to testify, too. I will attend the trial whether I testify or not. I have to be supportive of our friends."

"Let us go to sleep now. I know you are very tired."

"Thanks, Mom." Laura kissed her Mom good night.

The next morning, Laura did not get up until the phone rang. It was already ten o'clock. Debbie was on the other line.

"Laura, Mr. Bendle will meet us tomorrow at nine in the morning. Can you come to my office at eight?"

"That would be fine with me."

"Don't forget the two letters."

"I will put them inside my bag as soon as I hang up."

"I will see you at eight then. Take care, Laura."

"Thanks, Debbie"

By nine o'clock the next morning, Debbie and Laura were already talking to Mr. Bendle. Mr. Bendle took the two letters and opened them one at a time.

Dear Dr. Olsire,

Patty is going to report Robert Smith to the FBI office. He has to be stopped from abusing the homeless and from inflicting AIDS on the people of Philadelphia.

Thanks for everything,
Charlie Singleton

"Let's open the other letter, Mr. Bendle."

Dear Dr. Olsire,

My weakened mind and spirit awaited the arrival of Robert Smith every night. He would ask us to put out our needle-ravaged arms to make it easier for him to inject cocaine and at the same time to aspirate some blood with cocaine bank into the syringes. He was indeed a master injector. He performed cocaine injection and aspiration like an artist painting his masterpiece.

Two homeless people from my group died of AIDS before I got afflicted with it.

Please do something.

Thank you,
Charlie

"Mrs. Olsire, please leave these letters with me. I am going to get your copies authenticated now."

"We will wait for you, Mr. Bendle. Our trial will start April 27, 1986, at the Common Pleas Court on Market Street."

"We will send some undercover agents. Don't worry. We are not going to jeopardize your lives."

"Thank you, Mr. Bendle. You must realize that we have no idea whether members of the Sampaguita Cartel will be at the courthouse, too."

"We will post undercover agents near Smith's house. We have to know exactly how many of his men are around. Thank you for your cooperation, doctors. Keep in touch. Officer Eagle is working on this case with us, too."

Debbie and Laura drove back to Debbie's office.

"I can understand Patty's sudden change of attitude now. She is on a sting operation."

"I hope Robert Smith doesn't suspect her."

"I hope so, too. I have a sneaking suspicion that Euridis is an undercover FBI agent watching over Patty."

"I think so, too."

"We better be careful of the way we talk to or look at Patty. We will continue to ignore her if we see her. Otherwise, we will jeopardize her life."

"I know."

Laura went home directly after having lunch with Debbie. She passed by St. Archangel's Church to pray that everything would go well during the trial. Now that she knew the real scenario, the more she was worried. When she arrived home, she saw the sheriff waiting for her in the driveway.

Laura asked, "Is there anything I can do for you?"

"Yes," said the sheriff as he handed her a summons.

Laura thanked him and immediately ran upstairs. After she read the content of the summons, she started crying. Robert Smith had amended the lawsuit to include Michael's estate! He was suing her now!

She immediately phoned Debbie at work and told her what had happened.

Debbie said, "Don't worry, Laura. We'll get that shark sooner or later. While investigating him, I found out that his wife died five years ago. I then looked over the coroner's report in the investigation of the death of Linda Smith. I can't understand how he got acquitted of this crime! I just got in touch with the chief of the FBI in Miami. I'm going to send him a copy of this file; there is a similarity to the drowning case in Miami."

Two days before the trial, James Dillon and John Miller came to town. They both called Laura to see how she was holding up. She thanked both of them for their kindness and thoughtfulness.

On April 27, 1986, the trial of the first AIDS case in Philadelphia against four surgeons was about to start. Mrs. Patricia Singleton and her two daughters, Michelle and Kathleen, were the plaintiffs. The defendants were Drs. Jay Simmons, John Miller, James Dillon, and the estate of Dr. Michael Olsire.

The first day started with jury selection by the lawyers on both sides. This process took the whole day.

On April 28, 1986, the court crier announced the arrival of Judge Blumenthal. Judge Blumenthal called the trial to order. Judge Blumenthal called on both lawyers to give their opening statements.

Robert Smith, the sleek-haired, tall, muscular, and pompous plaintiff lawyer, gave his opening statement.

"I am here to present facts that Charlie Singleton was negligently transfused poorly-tested blood without his informed consent. As a result of the negligence of the doctors, he developed AIDS and died several months later."

Mr. Edward Sanborne made his opening remarks to the jury.

"I agree that Mr. Charlie Singleton was given blood transfusion, but this was the only recourse the doctors had to save his life. What Charlie Singleton had at the time of that emergency operation was a ruptured aberrant splenic blood vessel, a life-threatening situation."

Robert Smith called on Patty Singleton as the first witness who was sworn in to tell the truth and nothing but the truth.

Q: "Please, state your name and occupation."

A: "I am Patricia Singleton. I am a legal secretary."

Q: "How long had you been married to Charlie Singleton?"

A: "Twenty years."

Q: "How many children do you have?"

A: "Two."

Q: "Were you with Charlie Singleton the first time he was admitted to University Hospital?"

A: "No."

Q: "How did you find out that he was in the hospital?"

A: "Through my friend, Mrs. Fearless."

Q: "Were you upset when you found out that he was in the hospital?"

A: "Of course."

Q: "How did Mr. Charlie Singleton look the first time you saw him in the hospital?"

A: "He had gained about thirty pounds and looked older."

Q: "That is all, Mrs. Singleton."

Mr. Edward Sanborne came forward to cross-examine Patricia Singleton.

Q: "How many years were you married to Charlie Singleton?"

A: "Twenty years."

Q: "As you have stated a while ago, you were not with Mr. Charlie Singleton on January 9, 1983, when he was taken to the accident ward of University Hospital."

A: "No."

Q: "Were you home?"

A: "No."

Q: "Where were you?"

A: "At my mother's. I was living with her at that time."

Q: "Was Charlie Singleton living with you in your Mother's house?"

A: "No."

Robert Smith objected to the line of questioning. The Judge overruled the objection.

Mr. Sanborne continued, "How about your daughters, were they living with you?"

A: "Yes."

Q: "Where was Mr. Charlie Singleton living before he was brought to the accident ward?"

A: "The street in downtown Philadelphia."

Robert Smith objected again. Again, the judge overruled the objection.

Mr. Sanborne continued, "How did you find out he was in the hospital?"

A: "Through my friend, Mrs. Fearless, who was told by a police officer."

Q: "Why did this police officer approach Mrs. Fearless?"

A: "He was sent by Dr. Michael Olsire."

Q: "Did you talk to Dr. Olsire before you visited Mr. Charlie Singleton?"

A: "Yes, I did."

Q: "What did you think of him?"

A: "He was a nice person and a very caring physician."

When Patty gave this response, a startled Robert Smith gave her an angry look.

Q: "Did he help you in any other aspect of Charlie Singleton's care?"

A: "Yes, he went out of his way to help my whole family."

A furious Robert Smith loudly objected to Sanborne's line of questioning. After the judge overruled the objection, he sternly warned Smith to behave with proper court demeanor or he would cite him for contempt of court.

Q: "Do you think Dr. Michael Olsire was a good doctor?"

A: "He was an excellent doctor with a very good bedside manner."

Q: "Were you mad at Dr. Michael Olsire when your husband died?"

A: "No."

Q: "Was Michael Olsire taking care of Charlie Singleton at the time of his death?"

A: "No."

Q: "Who was taking care of him?"

A: "Dr. Tom Wittle."

Q: "Why was Dr. Michael Olsire still seeing Charlie Singleton?"

A: "Dr. Michael Olsire visited Charlie everyday because he had become friends with Charlie."

Q: "So you are suing your friend who is, himself, deceased?"

Patricia Singleton started sobbing and could not control herself. Robert Smith asked for a recess.

Robert Smith told Patty Singleton, Euridis, Kathy, and Michelle to go with him outside the court chamber.

"Patricia, what the hell are you trying to do? Were you testifying for the defense or for yourself?"

"I was testifying for the truth."

"Listen to me; anyone who does not follow my script will have her head blown away. This is not a threat but a promise."

Patty did not say a word but kept her cool. Euridis arched her brows. Kathy and Michelle were dumbfounded.

Robert Smith took Patty, Michelle, and Kathy back to the courtroom. Euridis stayed behind to make a phone call.

Judge Blumenthal called on Patty again for continued cross-examination by Edward Sanborne.

Q: "Do you think Dr. Tom Wittle took good care of Charlie Singleton?"

A: "Yes. Dr. Tom Wittle did his best in taking care of Charlie."

Q: "Do you know Dr. Jay Simmons, Dr. James Dillon, or Dr. John Miller?"

A: "No."

Q: "Do you know if they took care of Charlie Singleton?"

A: "No."

Q: "How come you are suing them?"

A: "My lawyer, Mr. Robert Smith, told me everyone involved in Charlie's care should be sued."

Q: "Do you know that Dr. Jay Simmons never touched or talked to Charlie Singleton and yet is being sued as well?"

Patty started sobbing. "I don't know anymore. I don't know why I am here."

Judge Blumenthal banged his gavel and called for adjournment of the trial.

On April 29, 1986, the next day, the trial started on time at ten in the morning.

Judge Blumenthal called the trial to order. He called on the plaintiff expert witness, Dr. Sam Greedy, to the stand. Robert Smith direct-examined Dr. Sam Greedy after he swore to tell the truth and nothing but the truth.

Q: "Please state your name and specialty."

A: "Dr. Sam Greedy; I am a pathologist."

Q: "How long have you been out of medical school?"

A: "Twenty-six years."

Q: "Are you familiar with the side effects of blood transfusion?"

A: "Yes."

Q: "What are the side effects of blood transfusion?"

A: "Hepatitis, Renal shutdown, Anaphylaxis, and AIDS."

Q: "Do you think Charlie Singleton's hepatitis and AIDS were definitely caused by blood transfusion?"

A: "Absolutely."

Q: "Do you think the four doctors should have taken precautions before Charlie Singleton was given blood transfusion?"

A: "Absolutely."

Mr. Sanborne objected to the leading questions of Robert Smith. Judge Blumenthal sustained the objection. After Robert Smith finished the direct examination of his own expert witness, Mr. Edward Sanborne stood up to cross-examine Dr. Sam Greedy.

Q: "Please state your name and address."
A: "Dr. Sam Greedy, 18 Sevilla St., Miami, Florida."
Q: "From what university did you graduate?"
A: "Florida University."
Q: "Where did you have your internship and residency training?"
A: "Florida University."
Q: "Are you in private practice? If so, how long have you been in private practice?"
A: "I am not in private practice."
Q: "What kind of residency training did you have?"
A: "Two years of pathology."
Q: "Are you board certified?"
A: "No."
Q: "Are you familiar with infectious diseases?"
A: "Not really."
Q: "What kind of infectious disease have you seen or treated during your training?"
A: "None."
Q: "How many times have you testified as an expert for Robert Smith?"
A: "One hundred fifty times."
Q: "Are you a hired gun?"
Robert Smith vigorously objected. This time, the objection was sustained.
Q: "Have you ever seen AIDS patients? Have you ever treated AIDS patients?"
A: "I have not seen or treated AIDS patients."
Q: "How can you testify as an expert of AIDS, when you have not seen a patient with AIDS?"
A: "I have read about AIDS in the medical journals."
Q: "When was the last time you had direct contact with any patient?"
A: "During my internship."
Q: "How long ago was that?"
A: "Twenty-five years ago."
Q: "Are you familiar with blood banks' operations?"
A: "No."
Q: "Do you know when the blood banks started testing for AIDS?"
A: "No."
Q: "Are you aware that, in 1983, blood was not being tested for AIDS?"
A: "No."
Q: "How could these doctors have taken precautions against AIDS when the blood bank industry was incapable of testing for AIDS at the time of Charlie Singleton's operations?"
A: "I don't know."
Q: "Would you call yourself a qualified expert of AIDS?"
A: "I cannot answer that."

Mr. Sanborne discontinued the cross-examination of Dr. Greedy. He approached Judge Blumenthal and in a low voice made a motion, "Your honor, I request that you declare a directed verdict. As you have heard, the testimony of Mrs. Patricia Singleton was practically a vindication of the defense. Today, we have Dr. Sam Greedy purporting to be an expert on AIDS when he has had no contact with a patient for twenty-five years."

The jury overheard Mr. Sanborne, looked at each other, and then eyed Robert Smith and Dr. Sam Greedy suspiciously.

"Let us recess for fifteen minutes. I want to talk to the lawyers of each party."

Patty Singleton, Euridis, Kathy, and Michelle left hurriedly. So did the FBI undercover agents.

Dr. Simmons got up to say hello to Debbie and Marguerite Dunn, but, all of a sudden, he stumbled and collapsed. James Dillon and John Miller quickly examined Dr. Simmons and tried to resuscitate him. James Dillon told Laura to call an ambulance. Debbie and Mrs. Dunn tried to get through the crowd that had surrounded Dr. Simmons.

Before the end of the recess, all the doctors and Mrs. Dunn had left with Dr. Simmons. The members of the jury told Edward Sanborne that Dr. Simmons had been rushed to University Hospital.

Dr. Simmons was rushed to a nearby university hospital. By the time they arrived at the emergency room, the EKG on Dr. Simmons was practically flat. Attempts to resuscitate him in the accident ward failed. Debbie was hysterical.

"I am going to get that shark no matter what it takes!"

Laura and Mrs. Dunn hugged Debbie and tried to console her. Both James Dillon and John Miller were in shock. They had just buried Michael Olsire six months ago! Both of them were in tears.

In the meantime, at the Common Pleas Court, Judge Blumenthal declared a directed verdict. He reprimanded Robert Smith for abusing the legal process. He was going to cite him for contempt of court and recommend to the Lawyers Disciplinary Board that he be disbarred.

Dr. Sam Greedy was told by Judge Blumenthal that he needed a good lawyer to defend him for perjury.

Edward Sanborne left hurriedly to go to the hospital where Dr. Simmons was taken. The members of the jury stayed out of curiosity.

All of a sudden, Robert Smith opened his attache and took out a thirty-eight revolver.

"Judge Blumenthal, you are now my hostage. Please, get on the loudspeaker and tell the other four judges in the building to stop the trials in their chambers. Instruct them to come to this courtroom and to bring the juries and bailiffs. Do it now and do it fast! Otherwise, I will blow out your brains."

Judge Blumenthal made the announcement on the loudspeaker.

"Sam, get the bailiffs' keys and lock all the elevators and escalators. Then, lock all the doors and windows of the building. After that, go to the men's room on this floor and look for the khaki bag I've hidden behind the big trash bins."

"What's in it, Robert?"

"Sawed off shotguns, pellet and dart guns, and grenades."

"Robert, have you lost your mind?"

"Do it or I will blow out your brains, too!"

After Sam did all that Robert Smith had demanded, he ran to the men's room and found the huge khaki bag. He then returned to the courtroom.

Robert Smith took out the contents of the huge khaki bag.

"What are you going to do now, Robert?"

"I am going to make an announcement on the loudspeaker that I have judges, bailiffs, and members of juries as hostages. I am going to demand a plane that will take us to the Pineapple Republic."

The police advised the public over the radio and T.V. to stay away from Center City. The city was under siege by a lunatic lawyer and a deranged doctor.

All of a sudden, it started to rain heavily. There were also thunderstorms and lightning.

"Robert, are you sure you want to take downtown Philadelphia as a hostage? Even God is telling us something with this weather!"

"When did you ever start believing in God, Sam? I thought money was your God?"

"Robert, you have to think logically. We will never get out of this courthouse alive! You can't blackmail the whole city!"

"Sam, I have lost everything. I am going to be disbarred and probably be countersued by these doctors. And, you are going to jail for perjury! We both know why I sued these doctors. We had to fool the authorities about our own activities. This lawsuit was a perfect alibi for us. Nobody would have suspected that we were involved with Charlie singleton's AIDS if we had won the case! But you blew it, you son of a bitch! Why didn't you say you had personally seen several AIDS cases?"

"I know, but everything was backfiring on us!"

The thunderstorms and lightning stopped.

Robert Smith talked on the loudspeaker. He told the chief of police to take him to the Pineapple Republic.

"We have to think about this," said the chief of police.

"Robert, the whole room is shaking! Look at the ceiling lights! My God, look at the building across the street! It looks ready to collapse! My God, Robert, God is warning us! Let us surrender and start a new life!"

"Knock it off, Sam. You got me into all this mess! You were the one who got me started on drug dealing and selling of human body parts."

"I did not force you, Robert."

"You love money, too, and the good life."

"You even killed your own wife when she tried to turn you in to the authorities!"

"I did not kill her. She drowned. It was an accident."

"Robert, let's give up. The whole building might collapse."

"I would rather die in an earthquake than surrender."

The judges and everyone looked at each other while the two greedy men aired their dirty laundry in public.

"Sam, the earthquake has stopped. It has been three hours since I demanded the plane! I am getting on that loudspeaker one last time! If I don't get the plane I want by five o'clock this afternoon, there will be a bloodbath in this courthouse!"

"Robert, how can you talk like that?"

"Shut up, Sam! I will include you in the bloodbath if you don't stop pestering me."

An hour later, Robert Smith was still ranting and raving. He heard noises on top of the roof of the courthouse.

"The stake-out cops are on the roof! They are going to attack us through the windows. You judges, Halstead, Holden, Binstein, and Powers! Get on the loudspeaker now! Tell the chief of police to get me that plane! Do it, now!!"

The four judges did not budge an inch. No sound was heard as Robert Smith, using the pellet and dart guns, killed all four. Blood, brain tissues, and intestinal contents splattered onto the green carpet. The admixture of red blood and green carpet grotesquely parodied a decorated Christmas tree.

Robert Smith bragged, "The number of shots each one of these judges received was dependent on the amount of money they used to get from my payroll."

"Robert, why did you do that?"

Instead of answering Sam Greedy, he started shooting at the five bailiffs.

Then he pointed the gun at Judge Blumenthal and shouted, "You caused all of this!"

"You did it to yourself, Robert Smith. You thought you could intimidate all doctors and payoff all judges. Well, you were dead wrong. I know why you killed these four judges, too. I know they were on your payroll. You were afraid that, if you went on trial, they would turn as state witnesses against you. Give it up, Robert Smith!"

BANG! BANG! BANG!

Judge Blumenthal toppled to the floor. The jury members felt helpless. They knew Judge Blumenthal was still alive.

Sam Greedy shouted, "You're crazy, Robert! What do you think you're doing?"

Robert Smith aimed the gun at Sam Greedy. Two loud shots echoed through the chamber. Sam Greedy fell lifeless to the floor.

When he realized what he had done, Robert Smith let the gun fall from his hands and cried, "What have I done? I shot my only friend! Sam! Sam! I did not mean it!"

Blood dripped like water from the two bullet wounds in Sam's heart. The dripping of blood eventually slowed down to a trickle as if the loose washer of a faucet had been tightened. Sam Greedy died the way he had lived. Just as he had bled the medical profession and liability insurance companies for so many years by giving manufactured medical testimonies, so now was it appropriate that he himself had bled to death.

In the meantime, a couple of stake-out cops had succeeded in getting through the court chambers. Robert Smith had become oblivious to what was going on. He put the gun into his mouth, but he had used up all the bullets on his friend, Sam. He then prepared to jump through the window. Some members of the jury stopped him and made a citizen's arrest. The stake-out cops reached the chamber and seized and handcuffed Robert Smith. Judge Blumenthal was rushed to a nearby university hospital.

Robert Smith was arrested and sent to Holmesburg prison with maximum security pending his trial.

One week later, a grand jury was convened by the federal prosecutor, Michael Sanchez. The grand jury indicted Robert Smith on ten counts of first degree murder, twenty-three counts of first degree homicide (inflicting AIDS on homeless people), illegal possession of firearms, drug trafficking, money laundering, and obstruction of justice.

Dr. Simmons was buried quietly in a private funeral. Debbie went back to work one week later. Laura continued her residency and moonlighting at Smithsvale Hospital. James Dillon and John Miller both went home after the funeral of Dr. Simmons. Mrs. Dunn continued to communicate with Laura and Debbie. They all planned to attend the trial of Robert Smith.

June 25, 1986, was a big day in Philadelphia. It marked the start of the criminal trial of the now infamous lawyer who had tried to take the city of Philadelphia hostage. Robert Smith hired the number one criminal lawyer in town, but the solid evidence against him was overwhelming. The prosecutor's witnesses were Patty Singleton, Euridis, and Judge Blumenthal, whose testimony was taped from his hospital bed. When Robert Smith saw Patty and Euridis in court, he thought he would die. The first witness for the prosecution to take the stand was Patty Singleton.

The prosecutor also showed the video of the drug warehouse in Robert Smith's office. It was located behind his revolving bookshelves. The jury members and the spectators saw some whitish powder heaped on the floor ready to be scooped into each of the plastic containers; they also saw boxes and boxes of already packed cocaine bags, boxes and boxes of money in denominations of 500 or 1,000 dollars, cases of rifles, pellet guns, dart guns, grenades, and a map of how money was laundered from one country to another. Another hidden map found in one of his legal books was a detailed plan on how the Sampaguita cartel planned to take over all the drug rings in Philadelphia. In another hidden book were the numbers of Robert Smith's bank accounts in Switzerland and the Pineapple Republic. His assets in Switzerland had already been frozen.

More evidence presented as Exhibits B, C, and D were the letters which Charlie had left to Patty and to Michael Olsire before he had died.

Exhibit E was the total number of AIDS victims which Laura and Debbie had compiled.

Exhibit F contained the one thousand hair specimens taken from homeless people and the results of the tests done on them and compiled by Debbie. All the hairs clipped were positive for Cocaine.

After all the prosecutor's evidence was presented, the plaintiff lawyer, Alvin Sandalwood, decided not to put Robert Smith on the stand. He pleaded guilty on all charges. He was given the death penalty and a fine of twenty million dollars on July 8, 1986, a day which saw the city of Philadelphia come to a standstill. Everyone flocked to the Federal Courthouse just to hear the punishment of the monster who had made downtown Philadelphia hostage for a few hours. People booed when they glimpsed Robert Smith as he was taken to death row at Graterford Prison.

The death penalty had not been executed in Pennsylvania since 1962. He would be number one on death row among 118 prison inmates.

Three months later, on October 1, 1986, Robert Smith was extradited to Florida. He was accused of five counts of murder, drug trafficking, money laundering, illegal selling of body parts, and illegal possession of firearms. He also hired the number one criminal trial lawyer in Florida. The prosecutor presented Ditas as its primary witness. She did not have a video, but she had a daily diary of what had transpired in the mansion from the time she had arrived to the time she was nabbed by the FBI agents. The FBI agents had their own video of body parts in Smith's frigidaire, the drug warehouse in the basement of his mansion, the boxes of firearms and cocaine, and the money in the basement. They also had videotaped the exhumed bodies of the four companions of Ditas and of the last model who had drowned in Miami Beach.

Two FBI agents went to Philadelphia to talk to Debbie in order to investigate the death of Robert Smith's wife. There was a lot of similarities: both had Valium and alcohol in their blood, and both had tested positive for cocaine in their hair.

On October 31, 1986, the jury gave a unanimous verdict of death penalty. He was also fined fifteen million. Smith's lawyer in Philadelphia appealed the death penalty conviction in the Supreme Court, but the justices refused to hear the case. The State of Pennsylvania agreed to let the state of Florida carry out the execution of the dangerous lawyer.

Robert Smith felt no remorse at all. The once arrogant and pompous lawyer who didn't care about anything but money and power found himself in a desperate position. He thought he was going to make a name for himself and at the same time cover-up his illegal activities. He thought the AIDS lawsuit would make him the Master AIDS Litigator in Philadelphia. But everything had backfired! He inadvertently had exposed his own web of deception to the public and to his profession! He became the King of Crime instead of the King of Tort! He also unexpectedly became a denizen of death row at Graterford Prison and ultimately a reluctant occupant of the electric chair in a penitentiary in Florida.

POSTSCRIPT

After Robert Smith's trial in Philadelphia was over, Patty Singleton, Michelle, and Kathy went on the Federal Witness Protection program. Patty and her girls visited Laura and her family before they left Philadelphia.

Euridis was transferred to another state FBI office beyond the reach of the Sampaguita cartel.

Debbie, Laura, and Mrs. Dunn attended the whole trial. Debbie and Laura sent the newspaper accounts of Robert Smith's trial in Philadelphia to James Dillon, John Miller, Jorge, and Estela.

Following the conviction of Robert Smith, the frivolous suit against the estate of Dr. Ryan Dunn was dropped. The plaintiff could not find any lawyer to take the case. Mrs. Marguerite Dunn hired the former prosecutor, Michael Sanchez, to sue the plaintiff for harassment, abuse of legal process, and defamation of reputation.

Judge Blumenthal survived the gunshot wounds and went back to the bench.

Following the sentencing of Robert Smith in Florida, Ditas also had to go on the Federal Witness Protection program. She could not go back to the Pineapple Republic because the Sampaguita cartel headquarters were located there.

ABOUT THE AUTHOR

A devoted practitioner of medicine and fervent advocate of patients' rights, Emerita T. Gueson graduated from the University of Santo Thomas in the Philippines.

In addition to interning at Germantown Hospital in Philadelphia, Dr. Gueson did her General Practice residency at Community General Hospital in Reading, Pa., and her Obstetrics-Gynecology and Gynecologic Pathology Residency at PGH in Philadelphia with rotation at three Philadelphia medical schools: Jefferson, Hahneman and Penn. In 1970, Dr. Gueson was a gynecological research consultant on HERPES SIMPLEX at the University of Penn Dental School. She was on house-staff at Lower Bucks Hospital in Bristol, Pa., in 1971 and, from 1972, has been on the staff of Nazareth Hospital in Philadelphia. She also joined the staff of Holy Redeemer Hospital in Meadowbrook, Pa., in 1984.

Dr. Gueson is a fellow of the American College of Obstetricians and Gynecologists and of the College of Physicians. She is a charter member of the Obstetricians/Gynecologists Prolife organization. She is a member of the Catholic Physicians Guild, AMA, the Philadelphia County Medical Society, Pennsylvania Medical Society, and Women Physicians and Surgeons. Also, as a board member of Physicians Who Care, a national organization of over 3,000 physicians, she has been extremely active in her tireless support of patients' rights and her relentless pursuit of quality health care within an environment of cost-containment.

Among the various publications Dr. Gueson has been listed in are The Who's Who of American Women, The World's Who's Who of Women, and Marquiz' Who's Who of Medical Specialists.

Dr. Gueson's articles have been published in the Journal of Reproductive Medicine, in the Philadelphia Daily News, Private Practice, and Physicians Who Care newsletter. Her first book, DOCTORS UNDER FIRE, was published in 1989 by Vantage Press.

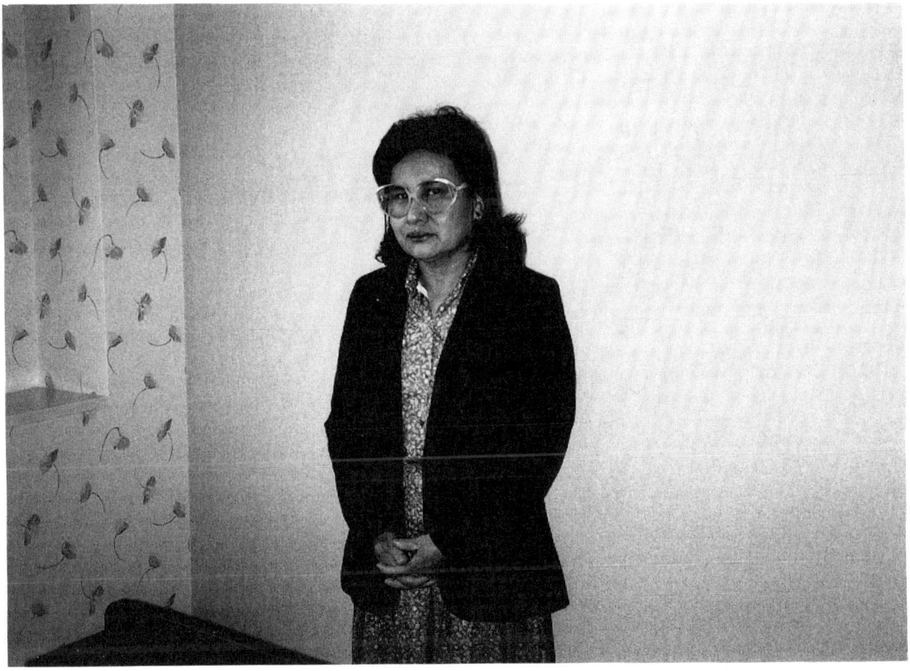